ADVANCED CRYSTAL THERAPEUTICS ^{sm}

by

Rev. Ojela Frank

Published by:

The Holistic Health Works
P.O. Box 327-AT
New City, N.Y. 10956   USA

Printed in the United States of America
by Riverrun Press of Piermont, New York

ISBN # 0-9619010-1-2

Library of Congress Catalog Number: # 88-081908

Cover and crystal illustrations by Michael McManus

Rose illustrations and calligraphy by Erica Risser-Runkles

Back Cover photo by Sal Cordaro

Crystal Therapeutics^{SM} is a division of Spiritual Awareness
Dynamics, Inc.

BOOKS by REV. OJELA FRANK

Crystal Therapeutics

Advanced Crystal Therapeutics

Crystal Therapeutics Teachers' Manual
(for certified teachers only)

This book is dedicated to all of those who

have the courage to find their Inner Light.

TABLE OF CONTENTS

ADVANCED TECHNIQUES with CRYSTALS for
CONNECTING with YOUR HIGHER SELF

OUR OWN PERSONAL TRINITY

HEALING

CRYSTAL HEALING MEDITATIONS

POTPOURRI

SPIRITUAL CLEANSING and RELEASING

THE HOLY SACRAMENTS and CRYSTALS

A WEDDING CEREMONY USING CRYSTALS

COLOR HEALING with CRYSTALS

****

ACKNOWLEDGMENTS

I am thankful of my soul, Omalya, for guiding and supporting me throughout this lifetime. My personality certainly has been a challenge to her while I struggled to find out who I was inside.

I wish to acknowledge the many people and teachers who influenced me and shared a part of themselves along my spiritual quest: my parents, Thomas and Marie McMahon; my kind grandmother, Mary McMahon; Hedel Vaughn Henry; Brenda Macaluso, a healing sister; Artie Yeatman and the family from his community.

I want to thank the following people who have shared Reiki in my life: Reiki Master, Patricia Ewing; Reiki Master, Carol Vidula Krum; and Reiki Grandmaster, Phyllis Lei Furumoto. It has been over five years that I have experienced this wondrous healing gift in my life.

I am thankful for experiencing the gift of MariEl Healing through Ethel Lombardi.

I am thankful for experiencing the gift of Shantira from Shantira Master, Rev. Gayle Clarity.

I am thankful for all of the crystal teachers who have shared with me in person, in their books or videos.

I especially want to thank Dr. Frank Alper of the Arizona Metaphysical Society. The Carousel of Growth Seminars were a great influence on me while I was writing this book. We thank you for your sharing, Adamis.

I again appreciate the support and editing from my friend, Eugene Frank.

I wish to thank my assistant, Helga Ottenberg, who offered her services to those clients whom I was unable to see because of my involvement in this book.

Thank you to my apprentices: Ann Romansky, Susan Chester, Mary Ryan, Regina Hugendubler and Connie Hanham. I appreciate your genuine, loving support and assistance in my business and at the workshops.

Thank you, Erica Risser-Runkles, for the beautiful rose illustrations and the calligraphy work.

I want to thank Michael McManus for his wonderful crystal illustrations.

I want to thank Donna and Stephen Schwartz of Riverrun Press for their support and guidance in helping me to produce my books.

I would like to thank Ben Buxton for taking an interest in my book, <u>Crystal Therapeutics</u>. Ben's interest and support inspired me to channel the personal color meditations.

Thank you, Dorian Caruso, for assisting in editing another one of my books. I appreciate your loving support.

Special thanks to Neil Borodkin and Joya Verde for the invigorating bodywork sessions and loving friendship.

I want to thank my national distributors, New Leaf, Bookpeople, Samuel Weiser, Inc., Wishing Well Distributing Co. and Starlite Distributors. Your support has made my dream a reality.

I also want to thank my regional distributors for sharing my books with their customers. Thanks to James George, Ingrid Smith, Artie Ford, Mandala Center Aum, Dave and Leonard Vukmanovich, Rev. Lamuel Salik, Riverrun Press and Sophia Tarila of the Crystal Coyote Co.

I wish to thank the Marcoulides family for asking me to do the christening for Malcolm and Alexander. It pushed me to go inward to come up with the ceremony for christening.

I also want to thank Elisabeth and Tom Baldwin for asking me to officiate at their wedding. Again, it was a catalyst for me to go inside to come up with a New Age style of wedding. I honestly feel that the ceremony will be used by many other couples as an outline for their weddings. We made history together. Thanks. It was great fun!

My appreciation goes out to Joan Hulse, one of my teachers in Pennsylvania. She taught me Thymo-Kinesiology and gave me the idea on the hand chart. I built upon it as my foundation in my healing work.

Thanks, Kimberly Conlon, for lending me a hand for my hand chart.

My heart goes out to all of my students who have supported me over the years.

My appreciation goes out to Mother Earth. Nature has quieted me enough to go inside. Thank you for the Colorado Rocky Mountains, the Black Hills of South Dakota and the Red Rocks of Sedona, Arizona. Thank you for the animal kingdom, the plant kingdom, and the mineral kingdom. This planet is very blessed.

DISCLAIMER

The healing crystals and products offered for sale by the author are not in themselves alleged to be a cure for any ailment, disorder or physical condition. Furthermore, it is not the intention of the author or the publisher to prescribe for any conditions, physical or otherwise. The manner in which this material is interpreted and used is the sole responsibility of the reader. We do recommend that you be involved in a well balanced diet and seek appropriate medical care as needed.

FOREWORD   by   Dr. Frank Alper

The Aquarian Age has thrust mankind into the world of crystals and magnetic energies. As each day passes, we become more aware of the increasing scope of our existence and the shrinking of the extremities of our universe.

During my recent travels throughout Scandinavia, Germany and Russia, I have found great interest pertaining to crystals already existing, as well as a strong thirst for more and more information and techniques.

As time shall pass, the general acceptance of crystals as legitimate tools for healing will become widespread. More members of the traditional healing practices are beginning to inquire, to study, and to utilize crystals in all forms of energy applications. The time will come when the integration of traditional and holistic healing will unite into one expression of service.

At this time, there have been many books written on the use of crystals. There can never be too many, for each teacher or channel correlates information from a different source and frequency. It becomes the responsibility of each reader to discern and to pick out the information that is compatible with his or her own individual expression.

Never allow your crystals to become a crutch for you to depend upon. Never use crystals as an excuse for your own lack of responsibility or confidence. Be responsible. Crystals are tools for you to use; that is all. They do not heal, nor do they perform miracles. Their sole function is to create energy fields. The rest is up to you.

In the following pages, you will find many wonderful explanations and techniques for crystal application. All of them are the truth of the author, for she is a responsible, dedicated person. You may not agree with all her truth, but if one point of information helps you to grow, she has served you well. Crystals are like wonderful children. They love to be touched and held. They enjoy the sun. They like to play with other crystals and generate love and energy.

I welcome you graciously to the world of the future as it emerges in the present.

Dr. Frank Alper

PREFACE

I have two spiritual children. They are my books, <u>Crystal Therapeutics</u> and <u>Advanced Crystal Therapeutics</u>. Each was created and carried inside of me for over a year. Each book is a labor of love. I have grown and evolved in the process of writing these books. They have been the reward for my efforts of journeying inward within myself. They are the jewels that I have found there.

The greatest catalyst for growth that I have experienced in this lifetime was my conscious connection with crystals. They have helped to accelerate my growth process tremendously. They are not my power objects. They are only tools. They are tools for growth. They are tools for amplifying consciousness.

My meditations began with quiet, solitary nature walks alone in nature. Other times, I would sit and look at a candle, or a picture of an ascended master, or a saint. Eventually, I was given a crystal and I wore it around my neck. Crystals found their way into my meditations. I would hold some. At other times, I would occasionally sit in a crystal grid pattern. Lastly, I began to hold a clear quartz sphere in my meditations. The whole evolving process developed over several years.

Each step of the way, my energy would be raised and my awareness would expand. I would awaken to a new level of seeing things more clearly. As I look back at this slow and steady process, I am thankful for all the teachings that came my way. Many people shared a part of themselves with me along my journey. I am thankful for our dancing, our interplaying together.

May the teachings that I share with you in this book help to support you in your awakening process. There is a spiritual door that leads to all knowingness. No one can open it for you except yourself.

Blessings in Light,

Rev. Ojela Frank

THE SWEAT

THE SWEAT 8/86

I am a child reborn
From the holy womb
Of Mother Earth,
Fearful, confused
And disoriented.

I see and feel
A new world
With new sensations
And yet, at the same time
There is numbness.

I sense new beginnings
Therefore, I do not know
What this will mean to me.

I can only trust.

I walk the Path
And know that the Great Spirit
Will take me
By the hand
And guide me.

I am reborn
And know
That all things are possible.

I am reborn
Within myself,
A merging
Has taken place.

I feel at one
Within myself.

I feel the power
Of who I am.

I feel the power
Of who I can be.

With my merging
Of myself
And with the Universe,
My inner power
Will grow.

1

PERSONAL   COLOR   MEDITATIONS

The following are personal meditations for many issues in your life. At different times in our lives, we all have areas that we need to look at and grow through. Use these meditations with or without a crystal and Angel Cards.   1.

These meditations are like New Age Prayers. Many are filled with affirmations. The words are just a basic formula to guide you through a particular issue. You can add to, or alter them as you wish.

You can use a quartz crystal along with these meditations. You can hold the crystal and say a meditation or affirmation. The crystal can be programmed with a personal meditation and the energy that was associated with the experience as you said it. You can carry the crystal around in a small pouch for a few days. This will act as a reminder of what you are selecting to change in your life. It will support you in your growth process.

These meditations, prayers and other exercises in this book are only tools. They are tools to assist you in your spiritual evolution. You will reach a level of being so familiar with these ceremonies, that they will become a part of you. One day, you will have evolved to a level of not needing to do many ceremonial procedures. There will come a time when you will think a thought, project that thought and it will manifest. We are all co-creators of the Universe. It is our birthright to know this.

1.   Angel Cards are a registered trademark of Kathy Tyler and Joy Drake.

4

Personal Color Meditation

Green:

Healing, balance, harmony and prosperity

Angel Cards: Angels of Healing, Balance, Harmony and Abundance.

I open to the color expression of green. It is the color of the Earth, healing, balance and prosperity.

I receive fully the color vibration of green into my energy field and into my being on all levels. (pause).

I call on the Angel of Healing to support me in my healing process. As I continue to grow and awaken, I release those unwanted, negative thoughts and emotions that have been accumulated over many years. I begin to purify my vessel. In this purging process, I ask for assistance of the Angel of Healing. I am open to healing on all levels of my being: spiritual, mental, emotional, etheric and physical. As this healing takes place, I begin to walk in balance.

I call on the Angels of Balance and Harmony. I am open to lessons that will teach me inner harmony. If I react with extreme measures in a situation, gently remind me of the scales of balance.

In the center of the balancing, I can focus on weighing and measuring both ends and all of the angles. I am in perfect balance.

Guide me with harmony so that I can overcome any inner turmoil that may surface at times. I am in harmony and balance. I am harmony and balance.

I call on the Angel of Prosperity, the Angel of Abundance. As a co-creator of the Universe, it is my birthright to have an abundant, fruitful life. I welcome prosperity and abundance into all areas of my life. I am open to thoughts and ideas that will help me to consciously manifest prosperity, in a constructive manner, in my life.

I am open to abundance. I am abundant. I am thankful for this abundance.

MY PERSONAL EXPERIENCE:

Personal   Color   Meditation

Blue:

Relaxation, overcoming stress, communication, expression, peace, patience and power.

Angel Cards: Angels of Peace, Patience, Communication, Truth and Power.

Quiet your mind. Breathe in relaxation. Allow your body to relax. Call on the <u>Angel of Peace</u> to come close to you and support you. Peace be unto you. Peace be with you. Peace be inside you. Peace be around you. Peace... you are peace.

As you fill your vessel with peace, it opens the way for patience. Call on the <u>Angel of Patience</u> to be near you and support you. The more peace you have inside you, the more patience you will have. Everything happens in its own course. As you adjust with the flow of what is occurring around you, patience will become a part of you.

The color blue activates the throat chakra, the center of communication and expression.

Call on the <u>Angels of Communication and Truth</u> to support you in expressing your true nature. As you open in your expression, know that others will be drawn to you. Walk in truth. Walk in openness. Others will do the same. When two or more are gathered in truth and openness, you have a blessed relationship.

As you walk in your Truth, you walk in Power. It is your guidance system. Call on the <u>Angel of Power</u> to come close to support you. Power comes from within, not from without. It is at the core of your being. Only you can give your power away. No one else can take it from you. Walk in your truth and you will always keep your power.

Affirm:
    " I am filled with peace. I have patience knowing that all things occur at their natural flow and pace. I communicate openness from my heart center. As I express my truth, I walk in power. "

7

MY PERSONAL EXPERIENCE:

Personal Color Meditation

White:

All of the colors combined together. A blending, a synthesis.

Angel Cards: Angels of Openness, Purification, Synthesis and Light.

     I am open to change. I am open to growth. I call forth the Angel of Openness to support me in my awakening to change. Change brings new beginnings and uncertainties. With my Angel's support I will have courage to face new things and change and grow inside.

     I call on the Angel of Purification. As I open, I release parts of myself that are no longer a part of whom I am becoming. Old memories, thoughts and feelings surface from inside of me. I clear away these energies. They have served their purpose. I have grown from experiencing them. I choose to let them go now. As I clear and release, my vessel is purified to receive more Light.

     I call on the Angel of Light to support me. I draw the angel's energies near. I have opened and cleansed myself so that I may receive greater Light. This healing, holy Light fills every level of my being. As a child of God, a child of Light, it is my birthright to receive this Divine Essence. I openly receive this healing Light now!

     I call forth the Angel of Synthesis. As I am filling up my vessel with Divine Light, I am blending with the Universe. I am becoming the Universe. I am one with the Universe. I am in perfect synthesis with all of Creation. I feel no separation. There is only completeness. I am one with everyone and everything. In this Divine Communion, I am the essence. I have become everything.

MY   PERSONAL   EXPERIENCE:

Personal   Color   Meditation

Pink:

Calming   emotions,   self-acceptance,   love,   compassion   and
forgiveness.

Angel Cards: Angels of Love, Compassion and Forgiveness

      I call on the Angel of Love for support in helping me to open
up fully to receive Love.   I am open to receive Divine Love into
every cell of my body.   My emotions become calm and in perfect
balance.   I fully receive love on every level of my being.

      As I open to the Divine expression of Love, I become one with
the Love Vibration.   I become Love expressed fully.   I am Love.
I fully accept myself for who and what I am at this present
moment.   As I love myself, I learn to express that feeling outward
to others.

      I call on the Angel of Compassion.   Teach me to have
compassion for myself and others.   Gently remind me to be easy on
myself.   My relationships will blossom as my heart expands with
compassion.

      I call on the Angel of Forgiveness to support me.   As I am
filled with love and compassion, I gain new strength to be a
forgiving person.   I forgive myself.   I forgive all others.
 For   give ... I give of myself.   I give to others.   I gently
remind myself that we are all human in nature. We are here on
this physical plane to learn and grow. This is school, a learning
process. Each situation, each relationship experience, enlightens
me one step further to an awakened consciousness.

      I walk my spiritual path in love, harmony and balance.

      I open my heart fully with compassion.

      For   give ... I give fully of myself in love.

MY PERSONAL EXPERIENCE:

Personal   Color   Meditation

Yellow / Gold:

Decision making, will power, overcoming depression

Angel Cards: Angels of Integrity, Joy and Power

    I call on the Angel of Integrity to support me in making
choices in my life. Gold is the color vibration of Spiritual
Wisdom. I gain this wisdom as I live in truth. I choose to live
my life in truth. As I am true to myself, I am true to others.
I am truth. I am truth expressed fully.

    I call on the Angel of Joy to assist me in seeing the many
blessings in my life. I am surrounded and filled with the yellow,
golden ray. It is the color of a big sunflower on a sunny day.
I welcome joy into my life. I feel uplifted with joy. I am joy.

    I call on the Angel of Power to guide me in my awareness. As
I become aware of who I am inside, I gain confidence and security.
I am aware of my center of will power. I will not let others
dominate me. Because I am secure within myself, I do not have a
need to control others.

            I am in balance.

    Because I live my life in truth, I have power. No one can
take my power away from me. Only I can let it go. Only I can
give it away to others.

            My life is filled with truth.

            I walk my life's path in truth.

            I am joyful as I count my many blessings.

    I am a powerful being. I feel my inner strength. I feel
secure within myself.

    Because my foundation is solid and strong, I have much to
share with others.

MY PERSONAL EXPERIENCE:

Personal Color Meditation

Purple:

Spiritual Attunement, cleansing, releasing, transmutation and healing.

Angel Cards: The Angel of Release and the Angel of Transformation

I call on the Angel of Release to come close to support me. As I awaken inside, a stirring takes place. Memories from the past begin to arise within me. Many thoughts and feelings come into my awareness. I recognize and see the many things that I have kept bottled up inside of me. They have remained buried deeply, so deeply that I would not have to look at them again.

I now understand, that for me to grow more consciously, I need to release the past. I ask for support in releasing all of my past, painful experiences. I am aware now that there were lessons I had to experience in all of those situations.

                 I RELEASE THE PAST.

I choose to grow from those lessons.

I am consciously processing all of these memories that come into my awareness.

I understand that the more I grow consciously, the more it is necessary for me to " clean my own house ".

" Physician heal thyself. "

" Metaphysician heal thyself. "

I am healing all the levels of my being as I consciously grow.

I am thankful for this releasing process.

As I release these energies out into the Universe, I call on the Angel of Transformation to draw near and to support me.

I am open to change. I am open to growth. I am open to transformation. I am open to transmutation.

15

I am being reborn inside. I am being renewed on all levels of my being.

I embrace this transforming process.

I AM RENEWED.

I AM NEW.

I have transformed to a new level of awareness.

I have transformed to a new level of awakening.

I AM AWAKENED.

I AM AWAKENED.

I AM AWAKENED.

I feel myself evolving each moment that I live. I am here to experience and to grow.

I am consciously evolving with each step that I take towards experience.

Experience is my conscious tool for growth.

Experience is my tool for transformation.

Each time that I grow more aware, I feel a deeper connection with my Inner Light.

Each time that I connect with my Inner Light, I sense an expanded awareness.

Each time that I sense an expanded awareness, I link up with Universal Consciousness.

When I am aware of Universal Consciousness, I feel connected with everyone and everything.

I become one with all.

I AM ALL.

I AM.

MY   PERSONAL   EXPERIENCE:

The Angel Cards used in these meditations were developed by two women, Kathy Tyler and Joy Drake, while living at the Findhorn Foundation, a New Age center in Scotland. They were originally designed as part of the board game called The Transformation Game. These Angel Cards are much more than just cards. They have an energy unto themselves.

I first came in contact with the Angel Cards through Reiki Master, Carol Krum. She had them spread out and faced down on the floor. Each class participant was guided through a meditation and then individually chose an Angel Card. I chose the Angel of Purpose. I called on the energies of the Angel of Purpose to come close to me. I could actually feel a presence of light energy next to me.

When you choose an Angel Card and acknowledge the angel's presence, those energies are amplified around you. Try it for yourself. If you cannot locate the Angel Cards at a local New Age bookstore in your area, drop us a line. We are a distributor for them. The Transformation Game is also available in some New Age stores.

I use the Angel Cards in most of my workshops. After each student has selected an angel for the day, I guide them through a meditation. It is an energy link-up process. Each student examines his / her card to see what angel was chosen. Each card has an angel doing an action that represents that particular energy. Example: The Angel of Clarity is looking out through a set of binoculars.

For the link-up process: Participants hold the selected Angel Card in their hands. They call on the energies of the angel to be near them. They hold the Angel Card in both hands and place them over the heart center. They make a heart connection.
(Pause).

Next, they hold the card at their throat area, the center of communication. They ask for assistance in expressing that energy outward to others. Next, they hold the card at their brow center and make an energy connection. Next, the card is held at the top of the head, the crown center. Lastly, the card is held at the Transpersonal Point (12" - 18" above the head) for the Universal Link-Up.

This link-up process amplifies the connection made with the angel's energies. You can also choose an angel for a person who is at a distance and in need of assistance. Just think of that particular person and choose an angel for them. Then send out those energies of support to that person.

I use the Angel Cards in Absentee Healing also. I may choose up to four angels for a person. I place each one around a photograph, at each of the Four Directions, or I may place an angel under a crystal on top of a signature of a person in need. Use your imagination. There are no limitations to healing work. Your intent is what counts.

CRYSTAL   and   GEMSTONE   ESSENCES

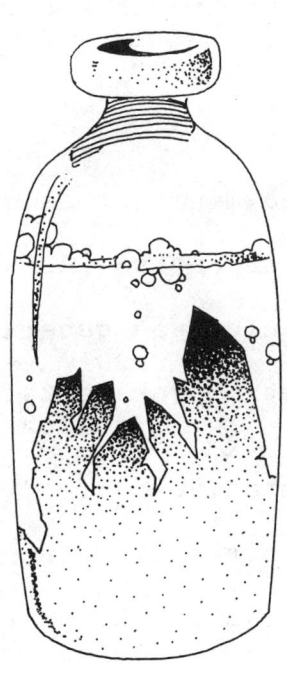

Crystal   and   Gemstone   Essences

Crystal essences have been used for thousands of years as powerful balancers. They aid in healing and reconstructing our physical, emotional, mental and spiritual bodies. Each of the following formulas contain the " mother " essence (first generation) to retain the highest color vibration from the minerals used. Each formula is uniquely different and contains the energy properties of a particular mineral.

Supplies needed: several gallons of distilled water; vodka; brandy; several glass measuring cups, 1 cup, 2 cup and 4 cup measurements; several gallon glass jars; several quart size glass jars; several glass casserole dishes; glass lids or cheesecloth; large rubber bands; coffee filter liners; funnels; empty dropper bottles, 1/2 oz. and 1 oz. sizes; labels.

When you begin making your essences, it is a good idea to have a few selected for basic needs. Here is a suggested list for starting out:

Rose Quartz - for calming and balancing the emotions.

Smoky Quartz - for grounding one's energy.

Emerald - Master Healer and general balancing.

Golden Citrine Quartz - for mental clarity, courage and
                                          for change.

Lapis Lazuli - meditative aid.

Amethyst Quartz - spiritual attunement.

Garnet or Ruby - for stimulation to overcome lethargy.

Many other stones can be used for gemstone essences later. Here are some suggestions for a secondary kit:

Aquamarine

Moonstone

Topaz

Tourmaline (pink, watermelon, or green)

Herkimer Diamond Quartz

Carnelian

Peridot

Celestite

You can use whatever stone you are guided to work with as an essence. Be careful to check out the chemical compositions of each mineral you are using in your essence mixtures. Some minerals are toxic and should not be taken orally. For example: Malachite, Azurite, Chrysocolla and Turquoise all contain copper. It is better to make a gemstone oil out of these, rather than to take them orally. You are making a vibrational therapy product whether it be a gemstone oil or an essence. As long as it is in one's energy field, it will be effective. Many people put drops of these energy products on their skin or in their bath water.

It is a personal decision for those who choose to take the essences orally. Some may feel guided to take four drops in their drinks three times a day. A good time to take essences is upon rising in the morning, before one goes to sleep at night and whenever it is convenient during the midday. Since you will be making the first generation, " mother essence ", it is recommended to dilute the mixture, if it is to be taken directly under the tongue. Or you can put drops of the mother essence directly in your drinks. Do not take the mother essence directly under the tongue; it is much too powerful. It is not meant to be taken in that manner.

The gemstone essences can be made stronger by putting them through different charging processes. Some can be placed under a pyramid for a few hours. Some can be placed outside under a full moon's light. Essences can be placed inside the center of a circle of quartz crystals. Use your imagination. Be creative!

Crystal and gemstone essences are effective the same way as flower essences. Have you heard of the Bach Flower remedies? Dr. Bach created them in England in the 1930's. They have over fifty years research now and are used all over the world by many doctors and health practitioners. The flower remedies represent the plant kingdom. The gemstone and crystal liquid essences represent the mineral kingdom. How do all of these essences work? They help to balance out one's emotional and mental state. Our physical condition also comes into balance. For example: What do you take to calm the nerves? Many people brew up some Chamomile tea or take the essence of Chamomile. That's support from the plant kingdom. Support from the mineral kingdom may come in the form of Lapis Lazuli. Essences help to heal the cause, not just the effect.

Be open to explore your own healing processes. These essences are tools for your growth. I see them as friends who are there to support my next venture forward.

If you choose to market the essences that you make, there are some addresses at the back of this chapter for products you will need. I manufactured Essences by Sá die successfully for four years. The essences have helped many and I appreciate the positive feedback I have received from many of my customers over the years.

I share with you now how I make my essences. I hope it is as rewarding for you as it has been for me.

Making   Your   Own   Gemstone   Essences

Cleanse the mineral of your choice.

Gather all of your supplies.

Pour distilled water into a glass container. You can use a glass casserole dish or a clean glass jar.

Put the mineral in the distilled water. Place the container out in the sun for at least three to five hours.

Place crystals around the crystal water mixture. You can have four large generator crystals at each of the Four Directions. Or you can place the mixture(s) in the center of a circle of crystals. The points would be aimed in toward the center.

If you have a large pyramid, you can put the crystals and mixture(s) in the center of the pyramid outside on a sunny day.

Noon time is a good time to begin the charging procedure.

Be sure to cover the mixture with a glass lid to keep out any flying particles and bugs. You can also use cheesecloth or keep the container uncovered and put the mixture through a filter later.

You can magnetize the crystal water by rubbing your hands together and placing them directly over the water for a few minutes. The energy flows out of your palm chakras and into the water.

You can also rotate a crystal pendulum clockwise over the crystal water for a few minutes.

The sun charges the water. The longer the mineral is in the water, the more the vibrational properties of the mineral are stored in the water. You may choose to charge the mineral and water together over a three day period, during the day time. Follow your inner guidance. Some mixtures may need to be charged under the sun and the full moon.

Once you have your charged mineral mixture, it is now time to add alcohol as a preservative. See the following mixture formulas for exact measurements.

Sometimes, the mineral mixture may get some debris in it. Use a coffee filter liner to strain out the mixture. You can use a quart jar and place the filter at the top with a slight indentation. Hold the filter in place by using a rubber band around the excess paper that overlaps at the rim of the jar. Pour the mixture through the filter liner slowly. When you have completely strained your mixture, remove the filter liner. Pour the strained mixture into a clean gallon jar. You are now ready to add alcohol to it. Decide if you want your mixture to be 100 proof or 80 proof. It is easier to work with a formula that has a 100 proof base.

Measure out your alcohol with a measuring cup. Pour it into the crystal mixture. For example: if you are making less than a 1/2 gallon formula, you would pour 15 ounces of vodka into 35 ounces of crystal water mixture. That gives you 50 ounces of an alcohol / crystal water mixture. You now have created the first generation " mother essences ".

When you are pouring more than one kind of essence during a processing session, always rinse out the measuring cup with boiling water. It's okay to use tap water from the sink as long, as you boil it. Next, swirl around a small amount of distilled water in the cup, to remove any drops of the boiled tap water. Each essence is a different vibration. If you do not rinse out each measuring cup as described, then you will carry one essence vibration into the next one that you are pouring.

You can place your essences in the sun, under the moon, or under a pyramid again. Whenever you feel guided to do so.

The next phase is to sterilize your dropper and empty bottles. Some people boil their droppers and bottles. If you choose to do this, be sure to have the glass products in the water before you boil them. Once they have reached a boiling point, lower the temperature gradually. If you take a glass product that is hot and put it under cold water, it will break. I rinse off the bottles and droppers with some running hot water from the faucet. Each bottle and dropper is done individually and then placed on a cookie sheet lined with paper towels. They are then placed in an oven at a very, low temperature. If you have the temperature too hot, it will melt the plastic caps of the droppers. If you have a gas oven, you can place the glass products in it overnight. You can heat the oven to 200 - 250 degrees, put in your rinsed bottles and droppers, and then turn off the heat. The pilot flame will keep the temperature in the oven warm enough.

Pour the gemstone essence out of the gallon jar into a measuring cup. Use a small glass measuring cup to pour directly into the small empty bottles. Add the dropper and draw a small amount of the essence into the dropper. Seal the lid tightly so that it does not leak. Be sure to label each essence correctly. It is easy to mix up the essences if you are producing more than one kind at a time. Do one essence, then go on to another. You can leave the excess essence mixture in the gallon jar. It will be kept for future use. I usually make up about twenty bottles of a particular essence at a time. When I need more, the excess is in the gallon jar. Figure out ahead of time what quantity you will need. I always make enough to last a season or two. In using the Sun Method, you can only make essences when you have the sun light. (Spring to Fall offers the best sun exposure for those who reside in Northern locations.) Remember that, if you are making large quantities to manufacture and sell to others.

You can charge your essences in the dropper bottles again at any time and in any manner that you choose. I say a prayer over each bottle of essence. I hold it in my hands and pray that the essence serve whoever is guided to take it, to his / her highest good.

You may be guided to add essences to your healing / counseling practice. I combine the gemstone essences with flower essences together at times. Each client's needs are different. Always leave the final choice of selection up to your client. You do not have a license to prescribe anything to a client who comes to you. You can counsel, hear you patient's needs and share what purpose each remedy is used for. The client makes the choice and most importantly, takes the responsibility for improving his / her health and life situation.

A few drops of essence can be poured into a shot glass of water. This mixture can then be placed over a photo of a person in need. It is a tool to aid others in absentee healing. I have experienced some amazing results doing this for those who have requested it.

Alcohol acts as a preservative and helps to maintain the subtle energy charge of the mineral into the water. If you want to <u>dilute</u> the mother essence formula, here is the procedure:

<u>Second generation</u> (stock bottle): Take two to five drops of the mother essence and put them into a dropper bottle filled with alcohol.

<u>Third generation</u> (dosage bottle): Take two to five drops from the stock bottle and put them into a dropper bottle filled with distilled water. Add 1/2 dropper of brandy for a preservative.

Follow your inner guidance as to what level of dosage to work with in taking the essences. It is okay to mix more than one mineral essence with another for your dosage bottle. Remember that if you choose to take directly from the mother essence, it's okay to put drops in your drinks, but do not take directly under the tongue. Some people put about two drops in their drinks. If it is a diluted mixture, it is okay to take directly under the tongue. Listen to your body. Ruby essence is very intense. It is a natural speed. It is very stimulating, so be careful not to do too much of it. Your body system will tell you what you need at times.

28

If clients come to you and they are totally against alcohol because they have cleared an alcoholic problem and may be active in an Alcoholics Anonymous group; they can use the essences on their skin, or in their bath. It is a vibrational therapy.

If you have been trained in Reiki Healing, MariEl Healing, Kofutu, Shantira, or any other healing art that uses sacred geometric symbols, you can etherically draw those symbols on the essence bottles to raise the vibrations of the essences. It really works!

You can purchase an ephemeris to examine productive times to charge the essences and / or crystals in the sun. If you are an astrologer, you will already know when it is a good time to do it. For those like myself, I picked up some valuable information in the book, Quartz Crystals and Other Gemstones. It states that one should not charge objects in the sun, when the Sun or Mercury is in any sign with 29 or 0 degrees. The author says that 26 degrees is a good time to charge objects. You can open the ephemeris to the month you are planning to charge your essences. Look over the columns for the Sun and Mercury. If you find 29 or 0 degrees listed, just skip those days. If you have an astrologer friend, he or she may be able to explain it better to you.

Essences can be taken at different strengths for various results. The following order lists the most effective to the least effective strength.

Orally: directly under the tongue from a diluted bottle.

Orally: a few drops in your drink from a diluted bottle.

Topically: a drop on your skin at the pulse points.

Topically: a few drops placed in your bath water.

Lastly, carrying around the essence bottle in your pocket. As long as the essence is in your energy field, it will affect you.

Gemstone Essence Formulas

1 cup = 8 ounces

1 pint = 16 ounces

1 quart = 32 ounces

1/2 gallon = 64 ounces

1 gallon = 128 ounces

32 ounces (4 cups)	30 ounces vodka
32 ounces (4 cups)	+ 70 ounces water
32 ounces (4 cups)	_____
+4 ounces (1/2 cup)	100 ounces
_____	
100 ounces	

100 Proof		80 Proof
30 oz. vodka	less	38 oz. brandy
70 oz. water **	than	62 oz. water**
_____	a	_____
100 oz.	gallon	100 oz.

----

100 Proof		80 Proof
15 oz. vodka	less	19 oz. brandy
35 oz. water **	than	31 oz. water**
	1/2	
_____		_____
50 oz.	gallon	50 oz.

----

100 Proof		80 Proof
7.5 oz. vodka	less	9.5 oz. brandy
17.5 oz. water **	than	15.5 oz. water**
	a	
_____		_____
25 oz.	quart	25 oz.

More   Gemstone   Formulas

<u>100   Proof</u>   <u>80   Proof</u>

3 oz.   vodka   less   3.8 oz.   brandy
7 oz.   water **   than   6.2 oz.   water**
_____   a   _____
10 oz.   pint   10 oz.

1.5 oz.   vodka   less   1.9 oz.   brandy
3.5 oz.   water **   than   3.1 oz.   water**
_____   a   _____
5 oz.   cup   5 oz.

**   The water listed in the formulas is the crystal water mixture
that has been sun charged.   Read the step by step directions
listed on the previous pages.   You will then see at what stage of
the processing you are to add the alcohol and create these
formulas.

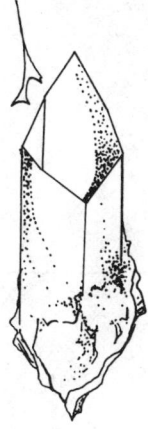

SAMPLE

Flow Chart for Manufacturing Essences

1st Day Process:
- Emerald ✓
- Golden Citrine ✓
- Amethyst ✓

✓ Sun Method: length of time ____3 hours____ (2 Days)
Mixture strained ✓
Alcohol added ✓
Mother Essence
Bottled ✓
Labeled ✓
Pyramid charge: length of time ____1 hR.____
Repeat Sun charge: length of time ____1 hR.____

-

2nd Day Process:
- Rose Quartz ✓
- Smoky Quartz ✓
- Lapis Lazuli ✓

✓ Sun Method: length of time ____3 hours____ (2 Days)
Mixture strained ✓
Alcohol added ✓
Mother Essence
Bottled ✓
Labeled ✓
Pyramid charge: length of time ____No____
Repeat Sun charge: length of time ____No____

-

3rd Day Process:
- Topaz ✓
- Tourmaline (green) ✓
- Aquamarine ✓

✓ Sun Method: length of time ____5 hours____
Mixture strained ✓
Alcohol added ✓
Mother Essence
Bottled ✓
Labeled ✓
Pyramid charge: length of time ____1 hR.____
Repeat Sun charge: length of time ____No____

32

Flow Chart for Manufacturing Essences

Day Process: Date & Time: _____
Essences:

_____   _____

_____   _____

_____   _____

Sun Method: length of time _____
Mixture strained
Alcohol added
Mother Essence
Bottled
Labeled
Pyramid charge: length of time _____
Repeat Sun charge: length of time _____

Day Process: Date & Time: _____
Essences:

_____   _____

_____   _____

_____   _____

Sun Method: length of time _____
Mixture strained
Alcohol added
Mother Essence
Bottled
Labeled
Pyramid charge: length of time _____
Repeat Sun charge: length of time _____

Additional notes:

Flow Chart for Manufacturing Essences

Day Process: Date & Time: _____
Essences:

_____   _____

_____   _____

_____   _____

Sun Method: length of time _____
Mixture strained
Alcohol added
Mother Essence
Bottled
Labeled
Pyramid charge: length of time _____
Repeat Sun charge: length of time _____

Day Process: Date & Time: _____
Essences:

_____   _____

_____   _____

_____   _____

Sun Method: length of time _____
Mixture strained
Alcohol added
Mother Essence
Bottled
Labeled
Pyramid charge: length of time _____
Repeat Sun charge: length of time _____

Additional notes:

Flow Chart for Manufacturing Essences

Day Process: Date & Time: _____
Essences:

_____   _____

_____   _____

_____   _____

Sun Method: length of time   _____
Mixture strained
Alcohol added
Mother Essence
Bottled
Labeled
Pyramid charge: length of time   _____
Repeat Sun charge: length of time   _____

Day Process: Date & Time: _____
Essences:

_____   _____

_____   _____

_____   _____

Sun Method: length of time   _____
Mixture strained
Alcohol added
Mother Essence
Bottled
Labeled
Pyramid charge: length of time   _____
Repeat Sun charge: length of time   _____

Additional notes:

ESSENCES   by   SÁ DIE

ROSE QUARTZ - Emotional healing, balances heart chakra for a loving disposition, self-acceptance. Calms upset emotional state, the " love " crystal.

RUBY - A natural stimulant (very powerful, a little goes a long way), increases energy level, activates root chakra, aids circulation, enhances courage, vitality and leadership.

AQUAMARINE - Peace, tranquility, meditative aid. Balances the throat chakra, opens intuition, the " vision stone ".

SMOKY QUARTZ - Aids in grounding one's energy when feeling scattered, emotionally upset, hyperactive or " spacey ". It also transforms on a more physical level, breaks up old patterns, cleanses aura, aids drug addiction pattern releasing.

TOURMALINE - (green) Balances polarity, realigns the mental bodies, helps to clear physical blockages, balances heart chakra.

EMERALD - Master balancer. Stimulates attunement to life force. Balances heart center, meridians and chakras.

TOPAZ - (Imperial Orange) Joy, lightness, expansion, creativity (artists), aids depression. Balances polarity and the solar plexus and spleen. Good for nervous exhaustion, tension and for " workaholics ". Allows the " child to come out and play ".

GOLDEN CITRINE - Mental clarity, focus, aligns lower chakras, in particular, solar plexus. Aids in raising one's consciousness, even if stubborn. Known as the " direction stone ", aids contemplation and finding a direction.

LAPIS LAZULI - Meditative aid, stimulates throat and brow chakras. The " initiate stone ", balances the mental body, aids the dream state, reduces inflammation.

AMETHYST - Spiritual attunement and transformation, cleansing agent, helps to transform old patterns and to attune to one's Higher Self. Aids alcoholism pattern releasing.

SUGILITE - (Royal Azel) Stimulates brow and crown chakras, balances the left and right brain hemispheres. Powerful aid for transition and transformation. (This powerful essence is to be used for dream state or meditation, not daily functions.)

Sources for Products and Supplies

Flower Essences

Bach Flower Remedies:

Ellon Bach USA (national distributor)
644 Merrick Rd.
Lynbrook, N.Y. 11563
(516) 593-2206

FES Flower Essence Society
P.O. Box 459
Nevada City, Ca. 95959
(916) 265-9163

Flower Essence Mixtures:

Santa Fe Flower Connection, Inc.
914 Baca Suite B
Santa Fe, N. Mex. 87502
(505) 984-1171

Flower Essences & Gemstone Elixirs:

Pegasus Products
P.O. Box 228
Boulder, Colo. 80306
(303) 442-0139

Flower Essences, Essential Oils, Energy Balancing Oils:

Star Child
The Courtyard, 2-4 High Street, Glastonbury,
Somerset, England BA69DU
phone: Glastonbury (0458) 34663

Crystal Essences:

Gemstoned, Inc.
2 Waverly Place
N.Y.C., N.Y. 10003
(212) 674-0970

Gem Tinctures:

Allachaquora
218 McKenzie St.
Santa Fe, N.M. 87501
(505) 988-9274

Gemstone & Crystal Liquid Essences, Attunement Oils:

Essences by Sa die

Holistic Health Works
P.O. Box 327, Dept. B2
New City, N.Y. 10956
(914) 634-2450

Oh Shinnah's Living Waters Series:

Little Turtle Trading Co.
3932 58th St.
Woodside, N.Y. 11377

Supplies:

Gilbreth International
3300 State Road
Bensalem, Pa. 19020

They offer plastic seals for glass bottles and shrinkable wraps
for shipping protection. You can use a blow dryer to shrink the
seal around the bottle top. You will need to send a sample of
your bottle. They will custom size seals for your bottles.

Empty glass bottles and droppers: (sold by the gross only)

Pennsylvania Glass Products Co.
429 Craig St.
Pittsburgh, Penna. 15213
(412) 621-2853

Roth Glass Co.
15 Wabash St.
Pittsburgh, Penna. 15220
(412) 921-2095
(Roth Glass Co. has cheaper prices than Penna. Glass.)

Continental Glass & Plastic
817 W. Cermak Road
Chicago, Ill. 60608

W. B. Bottle Supply Co.
836 E. Bay St.
Milwaukee, Wisc. 53207

Glass Funnels:

John M. Maris Co.
W. Main & Wall St.
Rockaway, N.J. 07866
(201) 625-2265

Perfume Bottles:

Carr-Lowrey Glass Co.
P.O. Box 356
Baltimore, Maryland

Plastic Containers:

Prescription Container
116-15 15th Ave.
College Point, N.Y. 113 56

Shipping Boxes:
U.S. Box Corp.
1294 McCarter Hwy.
Newark, N.J. 07104
(800) 221-0999

Plastic Boxes:
Bradley Enterprises, Inc.
450 T. E. Higgins Road
Elk Grove Village, Ill. 60007

Custom made labels and business stationary supplies:

NEBS New England Business Services, Inc.
500 Main St.
Groton, Mass. 01471

   For further information or to locate local sources, check your
phone book Yellow Pages. Another fine source for information is
your local library. Locate the Thomas' Registers. You will find
anything and everything in those books. They are reference books
that list products in alphabetical order.

Certification Training

Bach Flower Remedy Counselor

The Dr. Edward Bach Healing Society
644 Merrick Road
Lynbrook, N.Y. 11563
(516) 593-2206

Write for their national tour schedule.

FES Flower Essence Practitioner

Flower Essence Society
P.O. Box 459
Nevada City, Ca. 95959
(916) 265-9163

They offer practitioner's training at their center.

Essence Counseling Practitioner (flower and gemstone)

Spiritual Awareness Dynamics, Inc.
P.O. Box 596, Dept. B2
Bardonia, N.Y. 10954

LEARNING   HOW   TO   CHANNEL

Opening   Up

Just because you surround yourself with a bunch of rocks does not mean you will gain instant enlightenment.

It takes a lot of work to get to that place. It takes a lot of growth.

There are some short cuts to gaining a conscious awakening, but you still have to process and work through your own stuff that you've been carrying around inside your head for all of these years. You know, the stuff you always label others for doing to you. It's easier to blame others than to take the responsibility for ourselves.

I remember a lady calling me several years ago when I first moved to the New York area to begin my practice there. She had responded to one of my advertisements and called for further details. I still recall her conversation. She said, " You're not one of those people who think that you create your own reality are you? I can't relate to that. I don't believe it to be true. " I shared that I do feel that I create my own reality. She could not handle that realization and hung up the phone.

A turning point came in my life in 1976. I came across the book, A Handbook to Higher Consciousness by Ken Keyes. That book changed my life! Many of us are so busy trying to change others to our thinking, our ways. What we really need to be doing is changing our perspective of how we see the world, how we see others.   We need to let go of attachments and make them preferences. It takes a lot of energy out of us to walk around all day and be attached to every issue and everyone we are involved with in our lives. Thank You, Ken.

Energy follows thought. Even if you do not verbalize it, if you don't like someone that energy emanates around you. Here's an interesting exercise I learned from a Touch for Health instructor, Barbara Festa:

Gather three to five people together and line them up in a line. One of the end people will be your volunteer " tester ". You will muscle test that person. Have the " tester " raise his / her arm straight out. Test where it locks in place. Test for a " yes " and a " no " response just to get a feel of the difference. (This is important to do because everyone muscle tests differently and you'll need that comparison before doing anything else. Once you have muscle tested the " tester ", have everyone in the line connect their energies by holding hands. The person at the other end of the line opposite the " tester " will be the " igniter ".

Everyone else in between the two end people will be channels for the energy to flow through. They are to remain neutral throughout this exercise. You are now ready to begin: Go over to the igniter and whisper a negative statement in his / her ear. Something like, "I don't like the color of your shirt; it is an ugly color." Slowly walk down to the other end of the line giving the energy time to travel through the line. Muscle test the " tester ". You should get a negative response where the arm does not lock into position, it just drops. Return to the " igniter " once again. This time whisper a positive statement like, " I was mistaken. I really do like your shirt. You are a wonderful person. You have a beautiful soul. " Return to the other end of the line and muscle test the " tester ". This time his / her arm should lock into position for a yes / positive response.

What this exercise proves, if done correctly, is that energy follows thought. It also shows us how powerful our thoughts affect others. All of the people in the line did not hear what was whispered to the " igniter ". That energy traveled down the line and affected everyone else. Try this experiment. It can be a lot of fun and makes a powerful statement.

So, what I'm getting at is that we all need to become more aware of our thoughts and feelings. They affect us and others. They especially affect us and our health. Just think about that. When was the last time you had an intense, heated conversation with someone? How did it make you feel? How does your body react when you are angry with yourself or another person?

Several years ago, I went to a friend for a reading. It was a difficult period in my life. I had been going through an emotional upset for several weeks. This reader did not know anything about what I was going through at the time I had her do a Chakra Reading on me. She placed a hand in front of and behind each chakra center and tuned in to my energy. What she tapped into amazed me! I had become so emotionally involved in a situation with another person that it had completely affected my emotions, mental patterns, physical body and my chakra centers. Every one of them was out of balance.

One of my teachers during this same period began to notice that my energy field, my aura, was deteriorating over several weeks time. He took me aside and asked what was going on. He said that my aura was whitewashed.

I am sharing this information to remind you or alert you so that you don't get physically exhausted by allowing your ego and emotions to " trip you up. "

When you let go of ego and have control of your emotions, you find center. When you find center, you are able to channel more clearly and consciously through your vehicle.

The following is a sharing that I channeled to give to a group in Virginia Beach. As I began to understand these teachings, I saw the relation to a clean house, a clean channel. " Physician heal thyself. " The more you clear your own stuff, clean your own house, the deeper you go in and the more channels through you. You don't clearly channel unless your own stuff is out of the way. I hope that these teachings help you as they have helped me.

Healing Ourselves and Our Emotions

Each one of us is a spark. Each one of us is a Light... a light center.

We each need to ignite our flame and keep it shining brightly. At times, our lights may grow dim.

This occurs, when we lose our conscious connection to our inner light. When our focus is pulled outward by outside influences, in particular other people, this occurs.

Each person walking this earth has a dance...
lives a dance...
is a dance.

Look inside for a moment and ask yourself: " What is your particular dance? " (pause).

" What are you doing in life that makes you you? " (a long pause).

As we dance through life, some of our dances revolve around us; some revolve around others.

It is when we are at a moment in our lives revolving our dance around others that awareness or confusion may set in.

We dance. The other person dances and we both take on a new dance... together.

We each influence the other. Every person you meet in life influences you in one way or another.

When we are done dancing together with another person, when the dance is over, we have taken on a different dance.

46

It is important to share with others. That is one of the many ways that we grow inside.

        In our sharing...

        In our dancing...

We need to be aware of what part of the dance is our own, what part of the dance is the other person's, and what part of the dance or action is becoming... being taken on by the other.

Some people are aware of all of this.. Most people <u>are not</u>.

        So we dance through life
        Experiencing our own personal dance
        Meeting another
        Experiencing his / her own personal dance
        And then when we walk away...
        Are done being with that person,
        We have taken on and owned
        His / her own personal dance.

That can have negative, unhealthy results if a person has done this and is not aware of the pattern that has been created.

Another way to explain this is that some people are unconscious, unawakened beings. They are not in touch with who they really are and have not experienced who is inside them.

They are not only caught up in their dance, but for many, they also have the need to play " head games ". Their egos are weak. They have a low self-esteem. They are not in touch with their inner beauty or self worth. So, their dance includes, " mind games ".

How does this affect them? How does this affect us? An
example is will power. The dance of will power, the third chakra
is fully affected on both parties when this dance is played out
fully.

Power center: will, imbalanced

        manipulation

        domineering

        overbearing

        overpowering others

            vs.

        weak will

        weakened by allowing others to dominate us

        or control us.

    SEEK BALANCE.   SEEK BALANCE.   SEEK BALANCE.

Learning   to   Dance   Your   Own   Dance

     When you begin to get in contact with your Higher Self, it
occurs in stages. At first, it feels like someone else is inside
of you looking out through your eyes.

     You sense a gentleness all over your state of being, within
and without.

     When you are interacting with another " in the dance ", issues
may come up for you to look at and work through. A clearer
awareness is experienced as you go through processing emotional
issues that you need to deal with.

     A part of you is dealing with each emotion as it arises, and
you process it and clear it out. But, at that same time a part
of you is observing all of this interaction and knowing
consciously that this dance is not all there is to you. You are
much more.   Your emotions, especially unwanted thoughts and
feelings and pre-conceived ideas are all from past associations.
They are from past dances, past interplays with yourself and
others.

     The more one learns to dance his / her own dance, the more
conscious that person becomes. One has learned to drop past
associations and interplays.   One also learns to not take on
another's dance.

          How <u>Not</u> to Take on Another's Dance:

          <u>Finding one's own dance and dancing it.</u>

- Visualize a brilliant light within you. Center yourself in this
light. See and feel the light expanding outward and surrounding
you. Sense yourself walking in light.

- Know you are love and light.

- Seek to find a soul connection with the person with whom you are interacting. Know that beyond the dance the other is creating, he / she is love and light.

- As you sense your own light and love, be in your _present experience_. Be in your _now_ moment. Do not take your focus away from this; if you do, gently remind yourself to return your awareness back to the now moment. To do otherwise takes you out of the now. You run pictures in your mind of past associations or fears of the future that _you_ create. Ask yourself, " Am I projecting or experiencing ? " Projections take you out of the now moment. When you are consciously experiencing, you are active in the now moment.

As you are sensing your light and love and experiencing your _now_ moment, your channel will be gradually opened up. Your consciousness will expand into a greater awareness on how you see and experience life.

Let go of the issue of what's bothering you. Be aware that that is not your dance. It is either another person's dance or the interaction of both of you dancing together.

Stay in touch with your own dance, your own present moment. As you do this, your inner guidance will surface to your conscious mind. You'll be aware of your Light Connection.

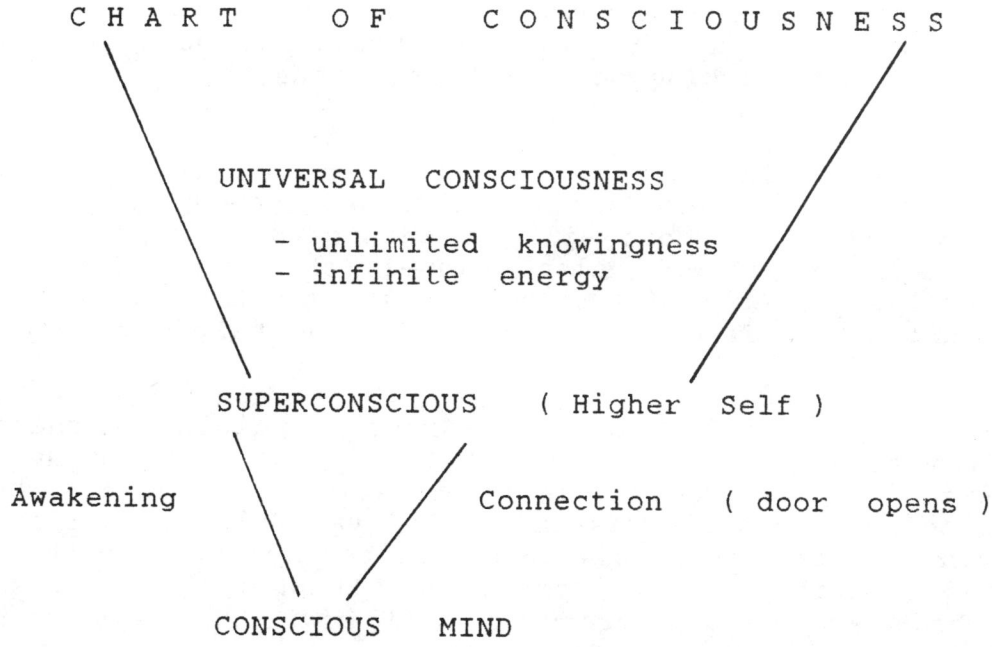

CHART OF CONSCIOUSNESS

UNIVERSAL CONSCIOUSNESS

- unlimited knowingness
- infinite energy

SUPERCONSCIOUS (Higher Self)

Awakening   Connection (door opens)

CONSCIOUS MIND

As you learn to go deeper in your meditations, you become more aware. Your vibration is raised and you are awakened to a new, higher level. Both your conscious and superconscious exist on an individual basis. As you awaken inside, the door to your superconscious (Higher Self) becomes opened and these two levels begin to blend together. It is here that you link up with an even higher connection, the Universal Consciousness. This all occurs in stages.

Little by little, you raise your vibration and awaken to a higher level. You bring these higher energies into your awareness. Many people sense these energies in physical manifestations. Some may feel " body rushes ", flashes, or energy surges; chills; or a sensation of being lightheaded. Another person may get a flying or floating sensation, as though a part of his / her self begins to lift out of his / her body. Another manifestation is a tightness or activity in the throat area for those who vocally channel.

Again, it is important to open up in stages so that you can adjust on the many levels that are involved in this process. Once you have consciously connected with the Universal Mind Consciousness, you have tapped into a magnificent reservoir of information. It is here that many are able to read the Akashic Records and learn about past lives.

When you consciously channel in your healing work, the supply source is unlimited. Energy just floods through you into the clients you are working on in your sessions.

The wealth of information you can tap into is tremendous. As you continue to raise your vibrations and open up, more knowledge will come to you. Most will be channeled through your Higher Self. Some people will also channel other soul vibrations and spiritual entities. Use common sense and discrimination about what information is given to you. If it is helpful, then use it.

See the list below for more advanced training in channeling. At this time, I only work with beginners. In my meditation practices, I have received many initiations by Spirit. They have been wonderful experiences and I feel very blessed. I feel that everyone who is consciously on his or her spiritual path can also experience this as well. Many of the techniques that I share in this book and in my workshops will give this opportunity to others.

Advanced training:

Dr. Frank Alper - the Carousel of Growth Seminars
Arizona Metaphysical Society, P.O. Box 44027,
Phoenix, Arizona 85064

Dan Baumgarten - channeling workshops: Dan Baumgarten,
West 444 23rd Ave., Spokane, Washington 99203

Sanaya Roman - channeling workshops: Luminessence Creations,
P.O. Box 19117, Oakland, Calif. 94619

Basic Video Tape: Complete Guide to Channeling (Assorted famous channels) $ 49.95 (We carry it.)

Audio Tape: Learning to Channel by Dr. Frank Alper
(Can be ordered through us, or the Ariz. Metaphysical group.)

Ken Carey (author of Starseed Transmissions) - channeling workshops: Ken Carey, Star Rte., Box 70, Mountain View, Missouri 65548

European Channeling Conferences: contact Dr. Frank Alper.

Common Sense About Channeling

Do not channel when your body is filled with alcohol or nonprescription, mind altering drugs. (You will attract only low, psychic vibrations.)

Do not channel when you are sleepy or tired.

We all have many voices inside our heads. Be discriminating about what you hear inside. Discern what is your true Inner Voice.

One needs to be relaxed, centered and focused to be able to channel.

Keep a note pad near by. This is good for those who have an overactive mind. You can write down thoughts as they come into your awareness. This is a good process if you are very creative and you keep coming up with ideas at the initial stages of your meditation. Once these ideas are written down, you can let them go and move on to a deeper level of your meditation that will open you for channeling. (If the distracting thoughts are about your relationships with others, or things that worry you, etc., then do the Pre-meditation Technique.)

Many people begin their channeling practice by writing down the information that they receive. Once they are comfortable with that process, then the next step is to use a tape recorder.
(You can purchase a lapel microphone at Radio Shack for less than $ 25.00. The voice softens for many who channel. Many times a built in condenser microphone will not record a loud enough volume level for you.)

Always review what you have channeled. Read your notes or play back the tapes.

Some people choose to channel only at their soul level. Others may choose to channel in addition to their soul, other spiritual energies. Each spiritual essence is unique and different. Some energies are intense and powerful, while others may be gentle, peaceful and so subtle that you may question if they are really there.

We can attune to each vibration on an individual basis. There is no limit to who you may be able to channel. No one has exclusive access to a particular soul vibration. As co-creators of the Universe, we can channel any soul or essence through us.

Channeling is like listening to the radio. You are in a particular mood and you want to listen to a certain type of music. You turn the dial from one station to another. In between each music station, you'll find a lot of static at times.

Each time we sit down to channel, our energy levels are different. We connect with a particular soul vibration. We listen and take in the teachings that are shared with us. We may choose to then move on and attune to another frequency, another soul energy.

As you loose your attention and focus, the energy link becomes weakened. It is like the radio dial got moved and you aren't hearing the music station clearly any more. There is much static. Tuning in takes focus. You must focus to keep in tune with the channel you are on. Many vibrations are so subtle that it takes more focus to keep the energy connection.

You do not need to strain your focus. In fact, if you apply too much effort, you will achieve nothing but get a headache in the process.

As you raise your vibration, the higher you go, the higher level you reach in connecting with another soul. That is why some channelers have more profound readings at one time compared to a reading they did at another time.

It will become easier to attune to your Higher Self or another soul's vibration after much practice.

If you are guided to channel past-life information in a reading, be careful what you share. Many people are misusing this information. I've seen several people use it as a " cop out ". They get information about themselves or another person whom they presently know and then manifest a karmic relationship based on the channeled information.

Do not become attached to those essences or energies you channel. If you do, you may find yourself bragging about it. That only involves ego. There is no room for ego in service work.

STARTERS

    Some suggestions for helping you to get started channeling are
as follows:

- Do readings for yourself.

- Practice writing down what comes through you.   Date your
material.

- Practice vocalizing what comes through you.   Use a tape
recorder. Don't feel threatened about this. You don't have to
play the tape for anyone else. Keep a collection of your tapes
and date them. It's nice to record your progress.

- Do a Chakra Self Reading: (10 - 20 minutes)
Hold your left hand over each chakra. Pause at a center until you
get an impression or a message relating to that area. Repeat the
process for each chakra center. Record what comes to you on a
tape recorder or make a mental note. Do not write down notes
while doing the chakra reading. It's too distracting.

- Do an Attunement Reading with photographs of friends and
relatives. The photo should only have one person in it. It is
too distracting to tune in to one person who is in a group
setting. Sense how that person feels. What impressions do you
get? Focus on the heart center. How does it feel? Happy? Sad?
Record your impressions. This is only for practice. Do not get
into doing a very personal reading on that person. This is just
an opportunity for you to learn to become sensitive from one
person's energy to another. Because it is done in private, it is
a comfortable exercise to do. Do not share what impressions you
get about another person. That is pushing yourself on another.
That is sharing unsolicited information. When the time is
appropriate, others may be guided to come to you for a sharing.

    Once you have gained confidence from successfully doing the
above mentioned exercises, then you are ready for the next step.

- Practice giving free readings to your friends and relatives. Mention to them that you have learned some new techniques and you would appreciate their support. Choose only those who are open to your doing this. This is a vulnerable time for you. If you give readings to those who are cynical or not supportive, they may upset you. This is a time to gain confidence through much practice. Some day you will be ready to go public.

When you are ready to go public about your channeling, you can do:

- Mini readings at psychic fairs.

- You can also offer to do channeling sessions for small groups. This can be done for a small fee or for free. As you gain confidence, you can channel for larger groups.

- Private Counseling / Channeling Sessions:

I put this one for last, because in a group session, readings can remain at a general level. Private sessions involve a deeper level of relating. It is a form of counseling. You are responsible for what is shared in this session. It is important to keep the communication open after the reading. This may be necessary for your client, if he / she is having a difficult time processing what you shared during the session.

Finally: When you are sharing a channeled reading with a client, it is important to stay in the now moment. Too many people are getting stuck in the past or the future. For the most part, I do not share past life information with those that I counsel. I do not channel predictions either. I have witnessed others doing prediction readings and that can be very damaging to those receiving the information. What I offer in channeled readings is guidance for the client. The teaching and sharing refers to lessons that one needs to look at in his / her life. Sometimes techniques are shared. These can help the client to deal with a particular situation that he / she is presently experiencing. Many times lessons and methods are channeled to assist one in accelerating his / her spiritual growth process. Be open to what you are guided to share. Don't get caught up in the past or the future. Flow with the NOW. The only limitations that you will experience are the ones that you create.

Channeling with Crystals

We are all channels. We all channel naturally, it's just that many are not aware that they are doing it. Inside of every person is an inner voice, an inner guidance system. We are tuning in to that place constantly. We judge, we select what is or is not good for us. Those decisions do not always come from past experiences or associations. Many times it goes way beyond that.

When I began to consciously channel, my first realization was that I had been doing it for quite some time. My gift of channeling has been experienced the strongest in my writings. I have always been a writer. It all flows so naturally for me. Some people channel on more of a vocal expression. Whether you channel in writings or by voice, the following exercises will open you up deeper than your present level.

Always begin these exercises with a prayer of protection. Set the condition that you are always in control. Be aware of your energy experiences and back down if you are experiencing too much too fast. It is always better to go slowly than to burn out by going too fast in your growing process.

Keep a pen and paper nearby for registering your thoughts and impressions. Some may prefer to use a tape recorder and vocalize the words as they surface.

As you become clear in your true expression, the door opens wide for wisdom to enter your awakened consciousness. Everything you will ever need to know is inside of you. It is your birthright to know this and to tap into it.

Blessings.

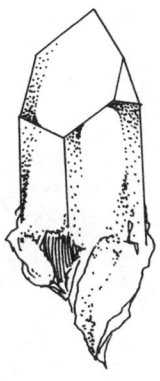

ADVANCED TECHNIQUES with CRYSTALS for
CONNECTING with YOUR HIGHER SELF

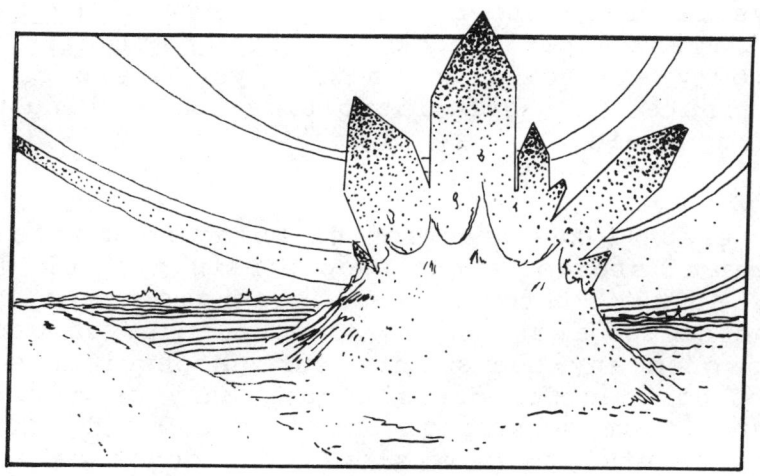

CRYSTAL BALL WORK

Quartz crystal spheres can be used for many purposes. Most are commonly used for looking into, also known as " scrying ". The energy of a sphere radiates 360 degrees. Quartz spheres are a powerful tool for healing and meditation practice. The following chapter includes many techniques for using spheres.

Warning: It is recommended that you do not attempt these exercises unless you have been meditating at an advanced level. These techniques will activate and awaken you to higher realms. If you are a beginner attempting these techniques, you may end up " blowing your circuits". Beginners are advised to do the exercises in my first book, Crystal Therapeutics. Also, many of the other exercises in this book will help to prepare you to reach an adequate level to handle sphere work.

It is recommended that you meditate without any crystals for at least a month or so. Then slowly introduce crystals into your meditation practice. You can begin by holding a crystal and continuing with your meditation routine. You can also meditate in a crystal grid pattern as suggested in Crystal Therapeutics, or in Dr. Frank Alper's book, Exploring Atlantis, Vol. I. Always begin slowly and build up to what you are capable of handling. Fifteen minutes is a safe intro time for working with crystals in your energy field.

The reason I keep mentioning being so careful is that I have heard several stories about people raising their kundalini energy up their spine (through their chakra centers). The ones who have done so too fast, have ended up in psych wards. We are not meant to open any doors into our unconsciousness until we are ready. That goes for drugs also. Many people have ended up in psych wards from " flipping out " on LSD and other psychedelics. Please be careful to grow slowly and don't take any short cuts. You may not be able to handle it.

I share with you the following techniques on activating yourself as a conscious channel. I do not take any responsibility for your processing it. It is up to you to take it all in consciously and slowly, a little at a time. I have given you ample warning. How you process this information is of your own doing.

Some people are more grounded than others. Those who are not will need to go at a slower pace. You may find it beneficial to have a friend or teacher with you, to assist you in these advanced meditations and be there for support. Be open to what feels right to you. As we raise the veil and have the opportunity to connect with our Higher Self, we have complete access to all knowingness. Take each session a little at a time and pace yourself. If you feel yourself getting too lightheaded or uncomfortable, then remove the crystals, or yourself from the crystal pattern. Each time you practice, you will build yourself up. As your energies come into communion with the energies of the crystals, you will meet a place where you balance out. Be aware at all times of what you are experiencing.

Always begin your session with a prayer of protection. There is a sample included in this book.

Some people who practice these techniques will begin to get in contact not only with their Higher Self, but their spirit guides. As long as you set the condition of protection and remain in control of what you are channeling, all will be fine. There are many spirit forms to tap into. Direct your focus to the highest level of Light that you are able to access and you will bypass lower vibrations.

On occasion, you may be exposed to a new spirit guide and find the energies are too powerful to connect with at that present moment. As you raise your consciousness and your vibration, you will meet those same energies more comfortably.

For example: I began to connect with a new guide. The energies were overwhelming at first. I would connect a little at a time. Over a six month period, I did a lot of growing on a conscious level. I then got the opportunity to visit the energy vortexes of Sedona, Arizona. While at Boynton Canyon, I connected with the same spirit guide as before. This time I was able to meet the energies on a comfortable level. I had raised my energies through conscious growth and this had affected my level of meditation and with what I was able to connect. It all relates.

An interesting thing happens when you practice meditation and begin to open up. Each time that you continue your practice, you pick up right where you left off. The crystals are only tools for getting you in touch with who you really are and what that consciously feels like to you.

As you reach a new level of awareness, the sensations may make you feel lightheaded at first. The next time you practice a crystal meditation technique, you may not need the crystal to reach that same level of energy and awareness. It is as if there is a signal inside of you that clicks into motion once it is triggered. A part of you remembers and acknowledges right where you left off. You are able to reach higher and higher levels of awakening.

The feeling of being lightheaded subsides as you become comfortable with sensing a raised level of awareness. Each day, you take it a little at a time so that you can remain comfortable with your growth process. You are adjusting. You are attuning. You are fine tuning your instrument and you don't learn this process overnight.

As you go deeper inside of yourself, many questions begin to get answered. " Who am I? " " What am I? " " Why am I here? " " What is my true purpose in this lifetime? "

You begin to take on a new understanding, a deeper relation to yourself, your life and your relationships with others. You open to channel light, love and peace. You blend into those sacred energies. You become light, love and peace. You are light, love and peace. Anything else that you acknowledge as being you is only secondary.

A Channeling Prayer

Divine Creator: Father, Mother, Son as One:

I ask for a blessing in receiving the healing Love Light of the
Universe. It is my birthright to receive this Light. I openly
receive this Divine Essence on every level of my being. I am
surrounded, filled and protected with this healing Love Light.
I call forth spiritual teachers of Light, spiritual guides,
Ascended Masters, beings of Light. I call these energies close
to me now. I ask them to support me in awakening and opening up
on a more conscious level. I open up the doorway to my Higher
Self, my soul. At this time, I ask for all of the teachings that
I need to look at, grow through and experience. I am open to all
lessons to be learned and sharings to be shared. I ask that all
of these things be brought into my awakened consciousness at this
time, so that I may verbally share them with myself and others.
I ask that this channeling come from my highest level of soul
connection. I ask that this channeling serve me and those here
with me to our highest good. It is good. It is done. So be it.

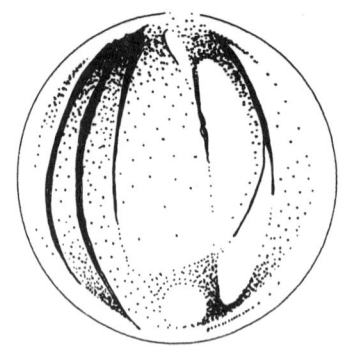

Crystal Ball Attunement

Supplies: One quartz crystal sphere.

          Two palm size crystals. Keep these within arm's reach
for the middle portion of this exercise.

Get in a relaxed position. Do the Relaxation Breath.

Be in a calm state of mind for five to ten minutes with your
crystal ball resting on your lap. Place both hands around the
quartz sphere.

When you feel you have relaxed and deepened your state of being,
then hold the crystal ball in both hands and place it directly in
front of the middle of your forehead (brow chakra). This will
begin to awaken energies in the third eye area. Stay in this
position for about three to five minutes. (It may be more
comfortable to brace your arms against your chest for support.)

Next, place the ball in both hands directly in the back of your
neck area (medulla oblongata, base of the skull). Hold the ball
in that location for three to five minutes. This is the energy
center that accesses channeling.

Place the ball in front of you with both hands at your throat
area. Hold the ball there for three minutes.

Place the ball over the thymus, then the heart, solar plexus, and
below the navel point. The ball is held in position in each of
these areas for three minutes.

Lie down and stretch out. Place the ball next to your coccyx
(root chakra). Support it with your hands. Keep the ball in
this area for 3 - 5 minutes, then remove it.

Continue lying down and place the ball on top of your chest area (heart chakra). Balance it so that it can stay there for a few minutes. Stretch out your arms at your sides. Make sure the ball stays on your chest comfortably. Take two crystals and place them in each hand. The crystal in the left hand is pointing up towards your shoulder. The crystal in the right hand is pointing down and away from your body. The heart center is the meeting point for the upper and lower chakras. " As above, so below. " Keep this position for five to ten minutes.

Stay stretched out and remove the crystals from each hand. Keep the ball on top of your chest area. Take your hands and place them over your face, covering your eyes and forehead. Continue relaxing and deepening your state of being.

When you feel complete, remove the ball from the chest area. Sit up <u>slowly</u> and go into a meditation for ten to twenty minutes without the crystals.

Sense how you feel and compare your sensations with what your usual meditative state is like. I found this exercise to be very powerful.

Alternatives:

1) One crystal in each hand at the heart chakra balancing it.

2) Turn the crystal ball counterclockwise, then clockwise, over the centers that feel blocked. Do this slowly and it will help to balance these areas.

MY PERSONAL EXPERIENCE:

Crystal Ball Meditation

Supplies:

One crystal sphere

Four palm size quartz crystals

One small phantom crystal or a " Herkimer Diamond " quartz crystal

Place the supplies within reach.

Place the four palm size crystals at the following locations:

1) left foot with the point up towards your body.

2) left hand with the point up towards your body.

3) right foot with the point away from your body.

4) right hand with the point away from your body.

Lie down and place the crystal sphere above your head.

Place the phantom crystal on your forehead at the brow center with the point up. You can use a Herkimer instead, if you choose.

Take some slow, deep breaths. Close your eyes and allow you body to relax.

Visualize yourself getting smaller and smaller. See yourself going inside the crystal on your forehead. Take a journey inside to see where it takes you....

When you are ready to return, bring your focus back to the room and your present moment. In a journal, write down your experience.

MY PERSONAL EXPERIENCE:

Crystal Ball Attunement with Amethyst

Supplies:

One quartz crystal sphere

One amethyst cluster 4" - 6" diameter

While in a seated position, place your left hand on top of an amethyst cluster. At the same time, place the crystal ball in your right hand and hold it over the solar plexus area. After about three minutes, the left hand may begin to feel heavy up to the shoulder / collarbone area. Switch by placing the right hand on the cluster and the left hand holding the crystal ball at the solar plexus area. Keep this position for another three minutes.

Next, place the amethyst at the feet, if seated in a chair; or at the calf areas, if seated on the floor. Place both hands on the crystal ball and hold it at the solar plexus for about three minutes.

Put down the crystal ball beside, or on top of the amethyst cluster. Keep both of them near your energy field.

Take the left hand and place it on the crown chakra. At the same time, place the right hand on the forehead.

Focus on opening your energies at these areas. Energy follows thought. (Pause for two minutes.)

Take the crystal ball and hold it against your chest with both hands over the heart center (about one minute).

Place the ball at the throat area for one minute.

Place the ball at the brow center for one minute.

Place the ball at the crown center for one minute.

Hold the ball at the Transpersonal Point (about 12" to 18" above the top of the head) for one minute.

Now, you are wide open for your personal meditation work.

On completion of your work, ground your energies and seal yourself in a bubble of light.

MY PERSONAL EXPERIENCE:

Advanced   Crystal   Meditation   with   a   Sphere

Supplies: a clear quartz sphere or a rutilated quartz sphere.

Hold a sphere at each of the following areas. Pause at each center with the sphere for about three minutes each. Say the following affirmations at each center.

Heart center: " I am open to love. "

Throat: " I am open to expression. "

Brow: " I am open to clarity. "

Crown: " I am open to spiritual growth. "

At 12 - 18 " above the head: " I connect fully to my Transpersonal Point. "

Hold the sphere over the 9th chakra (base of the skull): " I am open to inspiration and enlightenment. "

```
          I am open to Light.   I am Light.
          I am open to Truth.   I am Truth.
          I am open to Love.    I am Love.
          I am open to Peace.   I am Peace.
```

Connect both hands now to the sphere at the base of the skull and focus on this area. Energy will be concentrated in the area. If it becomes too intense, ground the energy by directing it down throughout your body.

First day: Do this connecting process for only three to five minutes. You may add a couple of minutes to each session as you become adjusted to the increase in your energy awareness.

Another addition to this opening process: You may also lie down with the crystal ball in your left hand and an elestial crystal at your throat area. Five minutes is enough time for the initial balancing.

If you feel guided, you may visualize a triangle or a cross on your forehead. These are sacred geometric patterns. You may know of another symbol and may choose to use that instead of these symbols. Follow your inner guidance.

MY   PERSONAL   EXPERIENCE:

Channel   Meditation

Supplies: one Elestial crystal

            one quartz sphere

Hold the Elestial crystal to the following areas:

    heart area

    throat area

    brow area

    crown area

    Transpersonal Point

    Medulla Oblongata (base of the skull)

After you have made a connection at all of the above centers, place the Elestial crystal at your feet. Hold a quartz sphere in both of your hands. You have " keyed " yourself in to raise your energy vibration. This will help you to reach higher realms in your meditations.

MY PERSONAL EXPERIENCE:

9th Chakra: Channeling Awakening

Supplies: a clear or rutilated quartz sphere
            a hand size, clear quartz crystal

Make an energy connection with each chakra for three minutes each.
Hold the sphere in both hands at the following areas:

- Brow
- Heart
- Throat
- Brow
- Crown
- Base of the skull

The right hand holds the sphere at the Medulla Oblongata (base
of the skull). At the same time, the left hand holds the crystal
at the Transpersonal Point about 12" - 18 " above the head:

Rotate the crystal in a counter clockwise direction for clearing.

Rotate the crystal in a clockwise circle seven times, while
descending downward to the crown chakra. When you have made the
seventh spiral, touch the crystal to the crown chakra and say the
affirmations:

        I am Love.

        I am Light.

        I am Compassion.

        I am Strength.

        I am Awakened.

Continue holding the sphere at the base of the skull with the
right hand. The left hand holds the crystal and touches it to the
brow chakra and you say:

        I am Awakened.

Take the crystal to the throat chakra and say:

        I am Awakened.

Take the crystal to the heart chakra and say:

        I am Awakened.

75

Take the crystal to the solar plexus chakra and say:

I am Awakened.

Take the crystal to the second chakra and say:

I am Awakened.

Take the crystal to the root chakra, at the base of the spine and say:

I am Awakened.

Zip yourself up with the crystal pointed at the second chakra. Move the crystal up to past each of the chakras and ending at the throat chakra and out.

While you are doing this, the sphere has been in position at the Medulla Oblongata with the right hand holding it in place.

Now hold the left hand and the crystal at the heart chakra. This is done at the same time, as the right hand holds the ball at the base of the skull.

Balance these areas; then remove the crystal from your heart center and sit with the sphere in both hands resting at your lap area.

Day 2: Same as above for connection process.

Additions: Do a clockwise spiral with the crystal in the left hand, while the right hand holds the sphere at the base of the skull. On completion, you can use both hands to rotate the sphere clockwise seven times at the Medulla Oblongata.

Day 3: Do not use the crystal point. Use the sphere starting with the base chakra and move it upward connecting with each chakra center. Follow through to the Transpersonal Point. Lie down and have the sphere at the Medulla Oblongata while meditating and vocalizing.

MY PERSONAL EXPERIENCE:

Focus   Charts

The following are charts for exercises in focusing. It is important to concentrate and focus in order to be an effective, conscious channel. Once you connect to higher energies of Light, it is important to not lose the connection. By using these focus charts and using other methods for focusing, you'll be able to hold the alignment longer.

My first official channeled session for a client was about ten minutes in length. When the woman returned a month later, the channeling lasted for one full hour. The difference was that I had a lot of practice in between the sessions. I built up my ability to keep the connection by using focusing techniques. Over a period of time, one becomes familiar with the sensation of connecting with higher energies.

How to focus:

There are several charts included here for focus exercises. Start with the first one. Look at the symbol for five minutes the first day. While you are looking at the symbol, think of nothing else. Just see and think about the symbol. If other thoughts enter into your awareness, just gently push them aside. Return to thinking of the symbol. When you have done the focus technique for five minutes, you are finished.

The next day, look at the next symbol on the following page. Look at it for five minutes. Do not think about anything else at this time. If other thoughts enter your mind, just gently let them go. Continue to look at and observe the symbol.

Day three: Look at the next symbol on the following page. Focus on it for five minutes.

Day four: Look at the next symbol on the following page. Focus on the symbol for five minutes.

Following days: Keep doing the focus technique for five minutes a day. Do this until you have gone through each of the symbols in the section.

The following week you will begin from the beginning again. Look at the first symbol. Increase your focus time to ten minutes. Do not think of anything else during this time. Each day you will focus on a new symbol for ten minutes a day.

The following week: Find a poster or a large photo of a nature scene. Make sure there are no people in the nature scene. Each day, set aside ten to fifteen minutes to focus on the nature scene. Look at it, observe it. During this time, think of only the nature scene. If other thoughts enter your mind, gently let them go. Continue this technique for three to five days.

The following week: Look at the nature scene. Project yourself into the picture. See yourself in the nature scene. Be there. Experience this for ten to fifteen minutes. Practice this for a few days.

The following week: Look at the nature scene for five minutes. Next, close your eyes to imagine the nature scene in your mind's eye. Explore the nature scene. If you lose a connection with the nature scene, open your eyes to observe the nature photo in front of you. When you have absorbed its beauty, close your eyes and visualize it again. Explore the nature scene. See yourself in nature.

Exercise   # 1:

Gather or purchase a small vase of flowers. Sit in front of the flowers. Focus on the flowers. See their beauty. Appreciate their beauty. Think of nothing else but the flowers for five to ten minutes.

Exercise   # 2:

Purchase or gather six to twelve red roses. Put paper and a pen near by. Sit in front of the roses. Look at the roses and appreciate their beauty. Roses are a very, spiritual flower. After you have looked at the roses for five to ten minutes, write a poem or thoughts about the roses. Open up to allow the words to flow through you and write them down. Read what you have written. (I wrote two writings about roses from a Quaker meeting that I attended.)

Exercise # 3:

Locate a tree with a large trunk. Take off your shoes. Embrace
the tree. You can stretch your arms around the trunk. Close your
eyes and take some slow, deep breaths. Plant your feet solidly
in the ground. Begin to feel a connection with Mother Earth.
Feel yourself becoming rooted into the earth. Be aware of the
life force of the tree. Sense the energy of the tree as you are
bonded to it. Allow your awareness to expand. Become one with
the energy of the tree. Sense how that feels to you.

Once you have linked up with the energy of the tree, allow your
awareness to expand. Feel yourself expanding and getting lighter.
Stretch your energy link with the area around the tree. Feel the
energies of the park or forest in which you are. Be aware of the
energies of everything that surrounds you. Become one with
everything that surrounds you. There is no separation. You are
one with everything.

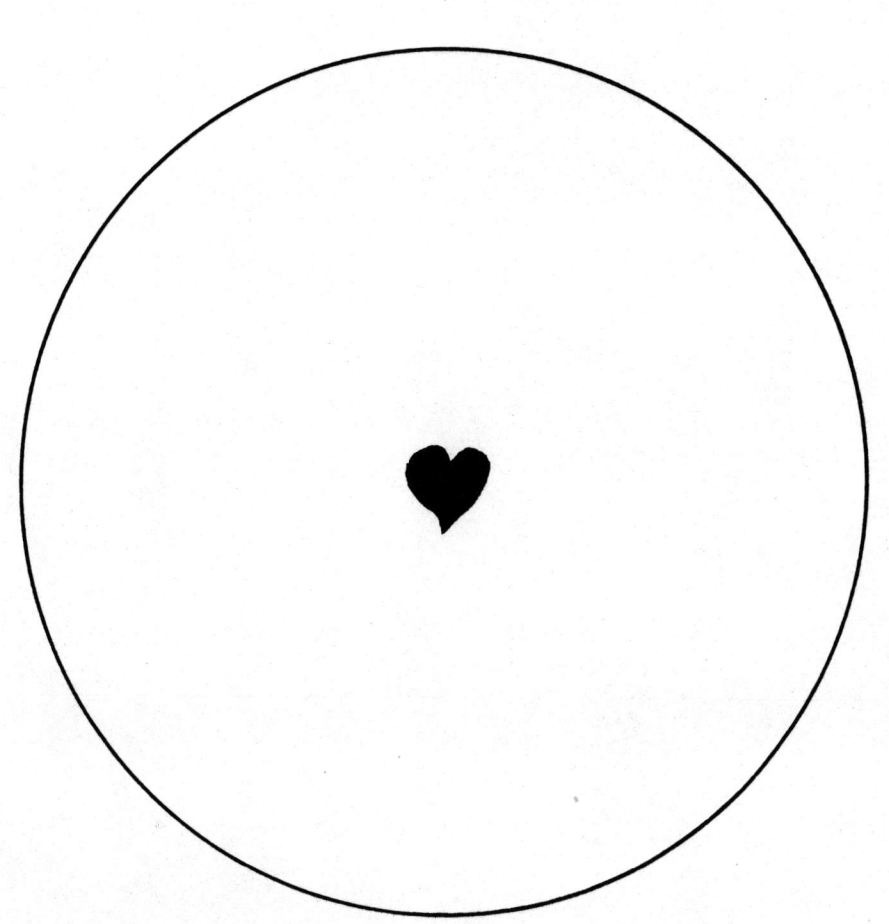

MY PERSONAL EXPERIENCE:

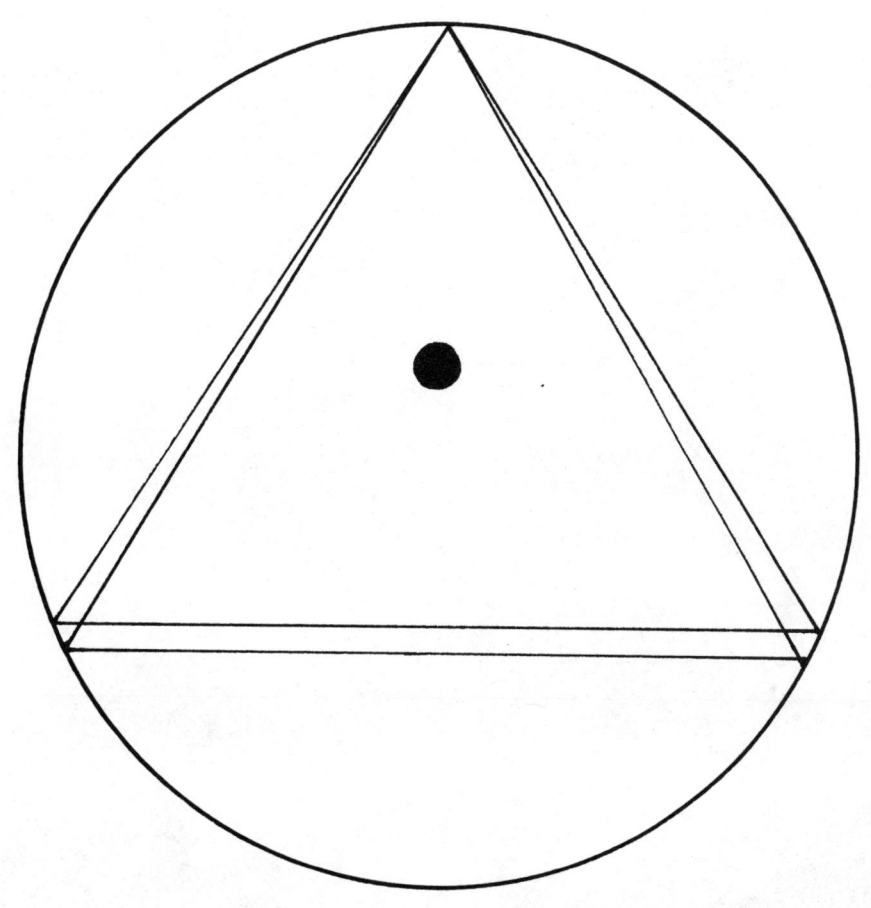

MY PERSONAL EXPERIENCE:

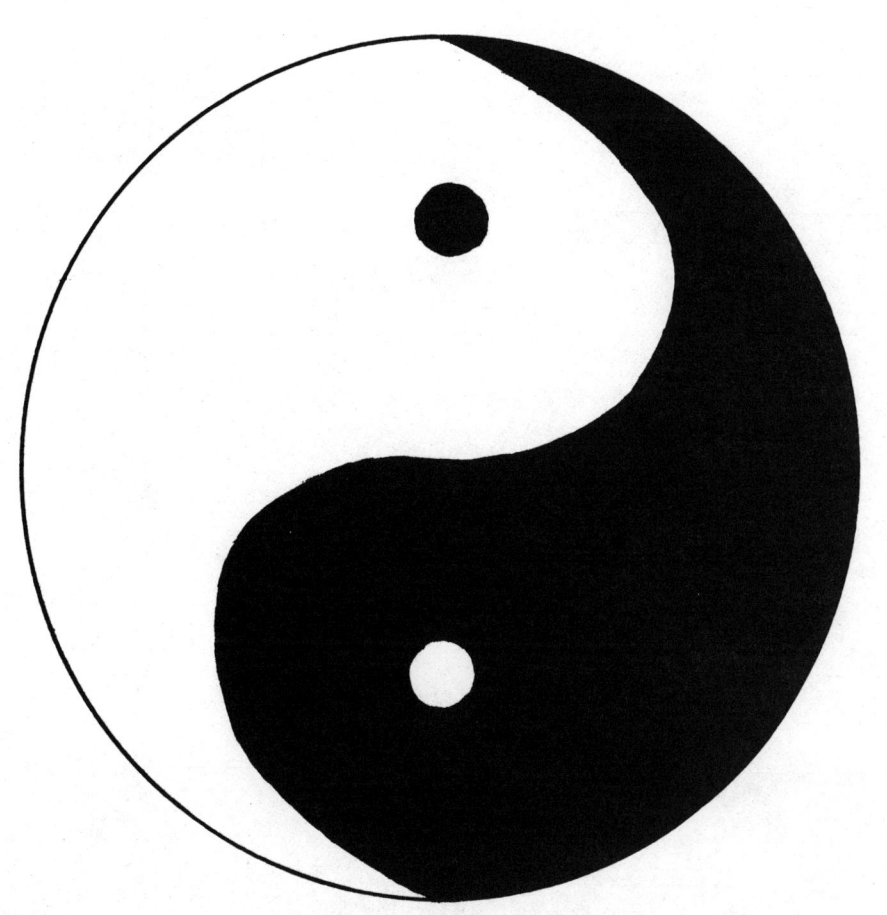

MY PERSONAL EXPERIENCE:

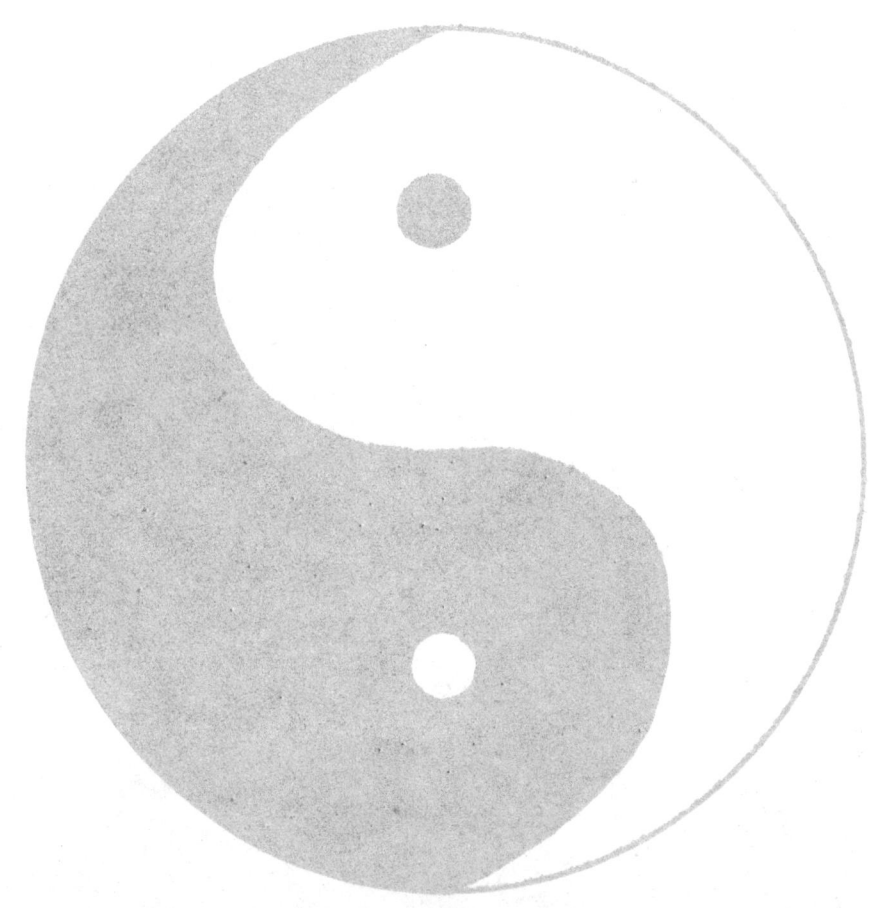

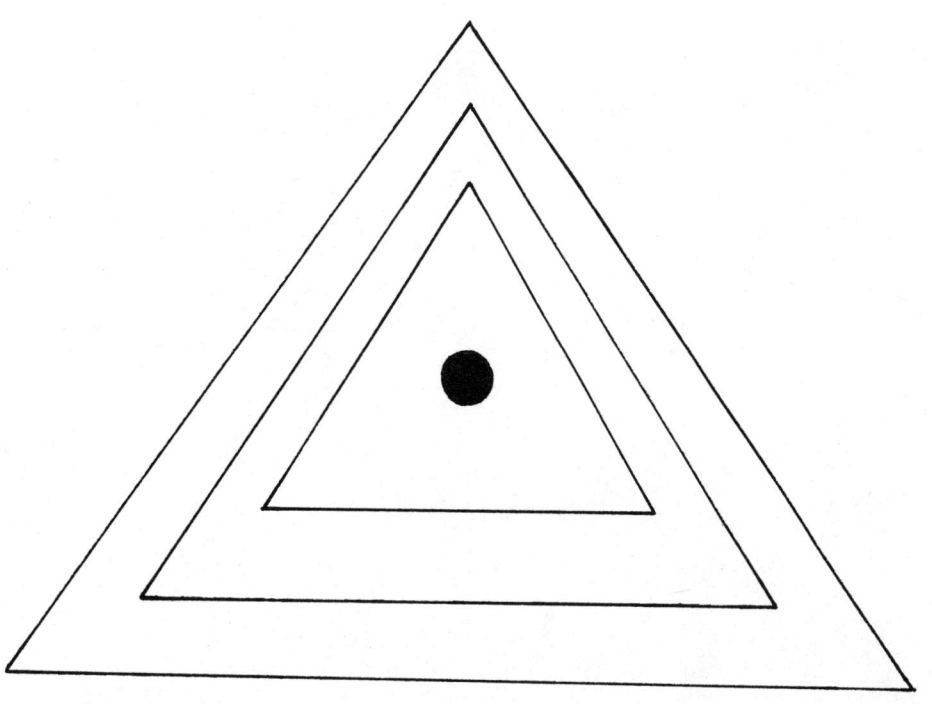

MY PERSONAL EXPERIENCE:

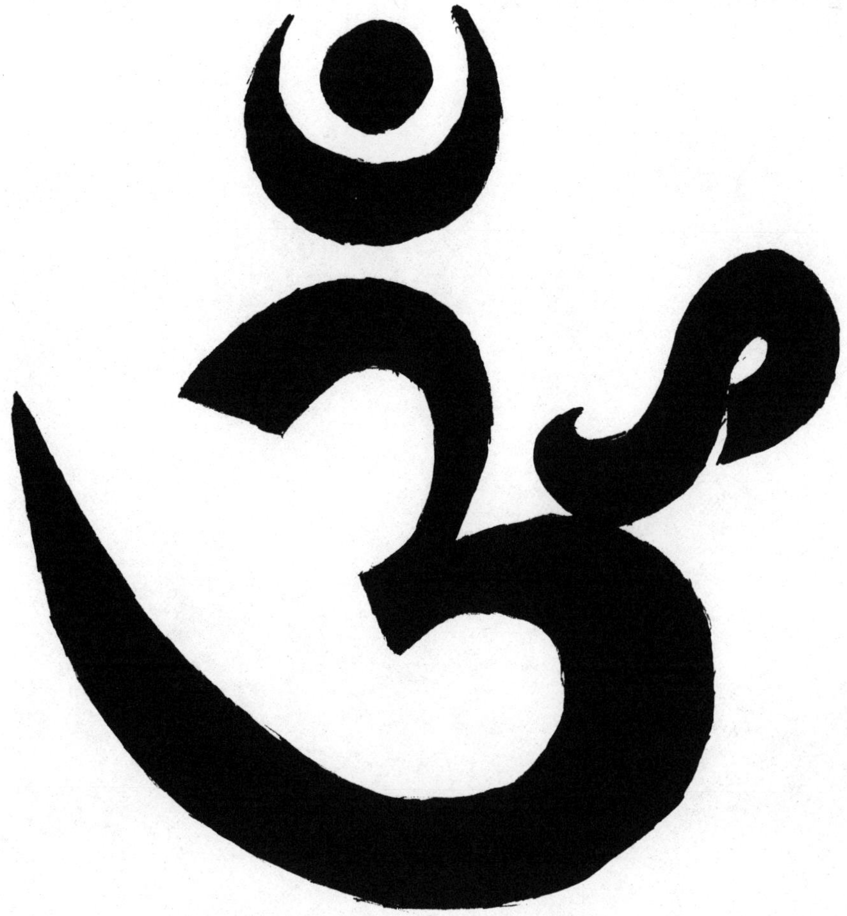

MY PERSONAL EXPERIENCE:

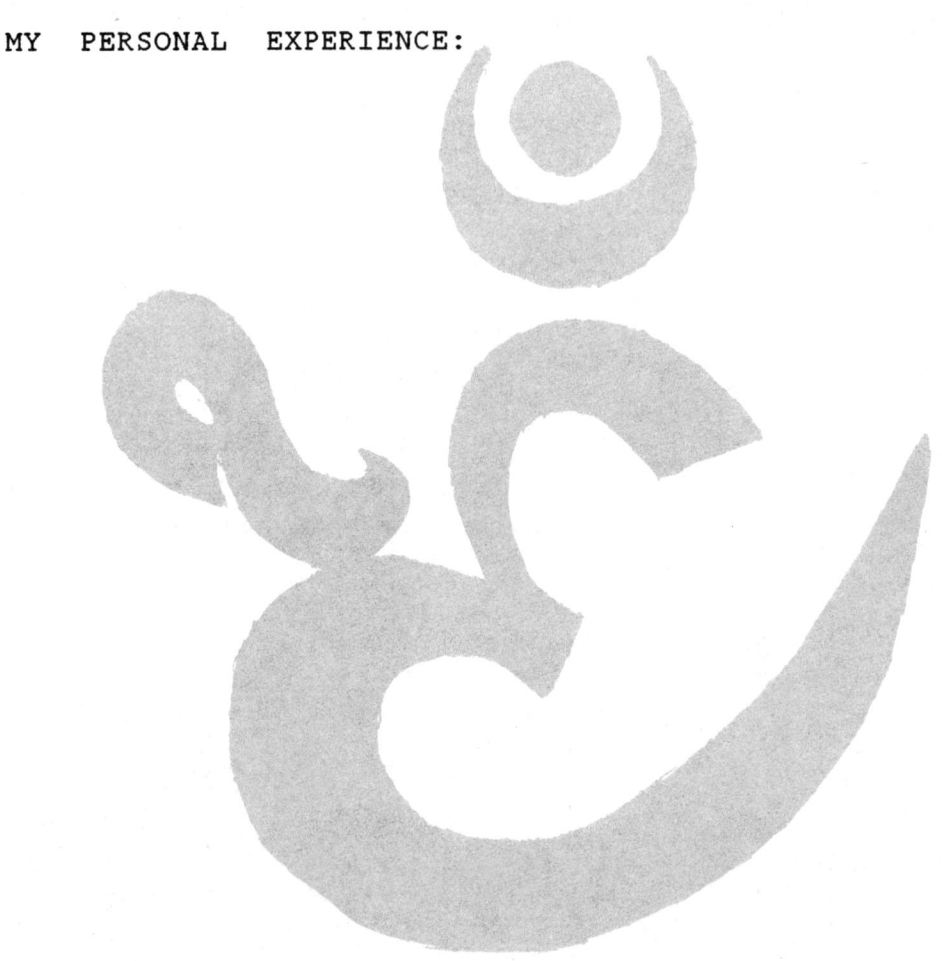

MINERALS   for   AWAKENING

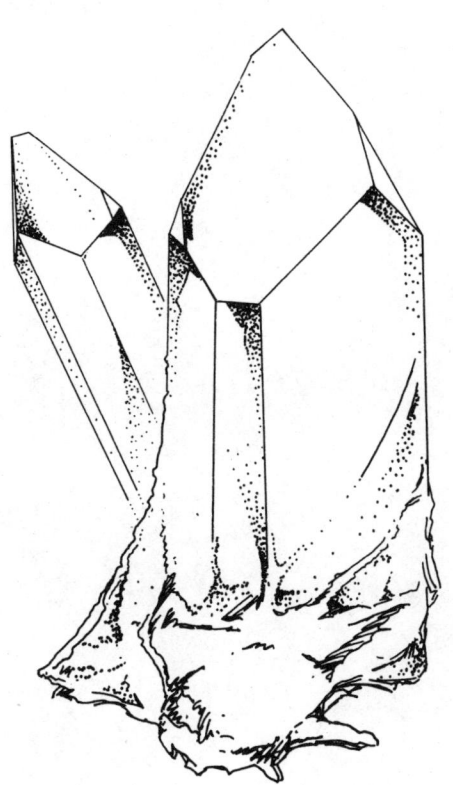

Awakening Your Inner Awareness and

Raising Your Conscious Vibration:

CELESTITE from Madagascar:

A couple of years ago, I went to have a channeled reading with Brian Dineen. When Brian and I sat down together, I noticed a beautiful cluster of crystals. The cluster was blue-grey color with gem quality translucence. I immediately was attracted to the cluster and asked if I could hold the mineral specimen during the channeling.

Brian began his channeled session and I held the celestite piece. As I began to relax, I became sensitive to the energies of the celestite. My energy became raised to a higher level. I began to feel lightheaded. A powerful presence could be felt by both Brian and me. I had made a connection with a new spirit guide. The energy link was overwhelming for me. I asked Brian what I had connected with. He tuned in and told me it was the energy vibration of an archangel! My body felt like it was buzzing all over. The connection was so powerful that I could feel the energy expanded throughout the entire room. Brian also confirmed this.

From this personal experience, I sensed that celestite was for celestial connections. To this day, it has been the most powerful stone for me to hold in my meditation work. I began to use it as a tool for connecting to higher realms. There are other celestites around from Ohio and Michigan, but there is no comparison to the energy of celestite from Madagascar. The rose quartz and clear quartz from Madagascar are also superb. Minerals from Madagascar are expensive.

ELESTIAL QUARTZ:

I first learned of this mineral in Katrina Raphaell's second book, Crystal Healing. When I came to the section on elestials, I skipped the information and just looked at the photos. I prefer to get my own personal impressions first, when sensing a new mineral. I located a six pound specimen at a mineral show. When I first held it, I got lightheaded and could feel a lot of shifting taking place in the upper chakra areas. I purchased the elestial cluster and took it home to work with it.

After the cluster was cleansed, I brought it to my meditation room. I was guided to stretch out for a meditation. (That was unusual for me. I usually meditate sitting up.) As I relaxed on the floor, I was guided to place the elestial near my heart area. I rested with it in that area for about ten minutes. It was a large, heavy piece, so I was on my side with the elestial in front of my heart. Once that area felt balanced out, I was guided to place the elestial in front of my throat area. I kept it there for ten minutes.

Next, I was guided to place the elestial in front of my brow chakra. I kept it there for ten minutes. Next, I was guided to place it at the top of my head to balance out the crown chakra. I kept it there for ten minutes.

On completion of this exploratory exercise, I was guided to hold the elestial in both hands and connect all of the chakras together. I held it over each center: the crown, brow, throat and heart chakras.

I was guided to place the elestial in my bedroom. I kept it near my head space for dreaming at night. During the mornings, I took the elestial to my meditation room. I meditated with it near my legs, as I sat in a yoga half-lotus position.

The elestial was with me in my alpha, theta and delta brain wave patterns for sleeping, or in meditation practice. I began to feel a shifting taking place inside of me. I began to grow consciously at an accelerated pace. I used the elestial as a tool for awakening to who I was. I began to practice linking up with my Higher Self. Once I adjusted to an awareness of higher frequencies, I began to consciously channel.

The elestial comes from Brazil. It is known as the "Jacare" crystal to the people from Brazil. I inquired about it at the Tucson Mineral Show. Some Brazilians were confused when I kept asking for elestials. When I asked for the Jacare (pronounced as Jock a ray) quartz, they knew what I was talking about.

94

SPHERES: See the section on : " Working with Spheres ".

SUGILITE:

   Also known as Royal Azel and Luvalite. According to Gurudas in Gem Elixirs and Vibrational Healing, sugilite balances the left and right hemispheres of the brain.   This is a very expensive mineral.   It comes from Africa.   It is usually sold by the gram.

   When I was first given sugilite to hold, I had a clue as to what it might do. It was medium dark purple. Purple balances the crown chakra. The piece I held was a very small cabochon about the size of a small finger nail. I placed it in my left hand. I immediately felt a rush of energy shoot up my arm. The focus of the energy occurred in the brow and crown chakras. A lot of activity took place there.

   I went to a mineral show in Virginia Beach last year.   I located a dealer who had a mineral I never saw before. There was nothing written on it either.   The mineral was charoite from Russia.   It was a medium, purple color similar to sugilite.

   At this show, I was talking to an expert wire wrapper named Peter Henry from Cincinnati. Peter had a cabochon of sugilite and another one of charoite. I asked if I could hold the charoite. As I tuned into the charoite, I could feel activity occurring in the crown chakra area.

   I then held the sugilite to compare the subtle differences to the charoite. There was a slight difference in the energies of both minerals.   I sensed that the sugilite was yang energy, masculine and powerful. The charoite was yin energy, feminine and more gentle.

   I was guided that both together would be a great balance for meditation work. I saw a meditation piece come into my awareness. It was a charoite cabochon on the left side and a sugilite cabochon on the right side.   I saw gold wire spiraling around silver wire. Charoite was in silver and sugilite was in gold. In the center of the piece was a small clear quartz crystal. The crystal was placed below the two cabochons to form a triangle. The crystal was pointing up. What a wonderful and powerful meditation piece. Maybe some New Age jeweler will make up this piece as described.

KYANITE: This medium to dark blue mineral is good for meditation work. It is also used for past life regression. I have used it with a few clients for balancing work and it helped to connect them with their spirit guides.

95

ENERGY PIECES: I come across many crystal practitioners in my workshops and at New Age exhibitions.   One thing I am beginning to see more frequently is powerful energy jewelry.   Last year, a student was taking a beginner workshop with me.   I noticed the woman was wearing a beautiful crystal pendant.   It was a Herkimer Diamond with a faceted moldavite.   I asked the woman if she wore the pendant frequently.   She said that she wore it all the time. The woman was new to working with crystals and I sensed that she needed to ground her energy.   I asked the woman if she had had any car accidents since she purchased the crystal pendant.   She thought about it for a brief moment and then remembered that she did have a car accident a few months ago.

   I told her that Herkimer Diamond quartz crystals are used for dreaming and meditation work.   They are used particularly for " out of body " experiences.   The moldavite is a green, glassy meteorite (tektite) from outer space.   Millions of years ago, it fell into a river in Czechoslovakia.   Many advanced students of meditation use moldavite for inter-dimensional and extra-terrestrial communication.   It was obvious for me to make the connection between the woman's crystal piece and her car accident. As the woman recalled her accident, she said that she was not totally alert and aware.   The crystal power piece clouded this woman's perception and made her lightheaded and " spacey ".   Over a period of time, the woman learned about energy work and became more grounded.

   A friend came to visit me the other day.   She was wearing a lovely jewelry pendant.   It was fashioned from a piece of polished sugilite with a faceted moldavite mounted on the top.   I asked her when she had purchased the pendant.   She bought it earlier in the day.   I asked her if she had driven while wearing the powerful energy piece.   She said she had driven only for a short period of time.   I asked her if she had come close to having a car accident that day.   She said that within one minute of driving her car from the crystal store, she had come close to being in a car accident.

   I want to make a point here.   I feel it is important to get this information out to the public.   I share information about wearing power pieces in my workshops.   While writing this book, I came across many others wearing power pieces.   This was a clear signal to me that I should mention a caution about wearing power pieces in this book.

   Power pieces are to be worn during meditation, ceremony or when in a dream state.   It is not appropriate to carry or wear powerful energy pieces while driving a car, flying an airplane, or operating machinery.   Most of the power pieces are for activating the upper chakras.   This helps to raise one's energy vibration.   It could be detrimental to their health, if people are not grounded and focused on what is taking place in their present moment.   Use common sense and stay alert.

As you grow within,
you grow without.
Your Light sparkles
through you to others.
You are a Light keeper.

As you are in perfect balance,
that energy emanates to others.
They in turn are affected.
They in turn come into balance.
Their Light sparks become
ignited and they share
their Light with others.

As our Light flames unite,
the World becomes a nicer place.
The World comes into balance.
The World becomes many
individualized Lights.
The World becomes one
great, big Light center.

From your center
to the World center.
The torch is carried
and shared.

OUR   OWN   PERSONAL   TRINITY

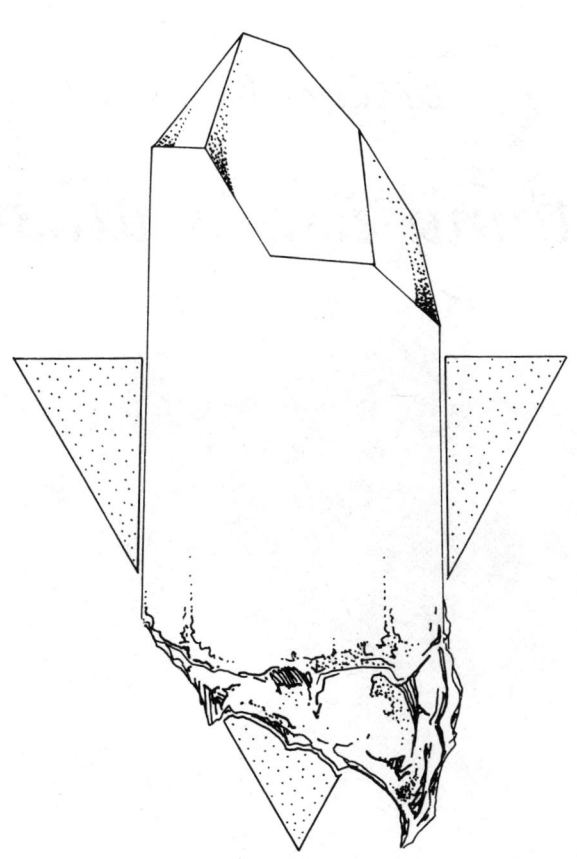

There is no separateness.

There is only expansion.

Anything else is illusion.

OMALYA

Our Own Personal Trinity

Each one of us has many facets that make up who we are. The followers of the great philosopher, Rudolf Steiner (Anthroposophy) refer to two trinities in his teachings:

1) Thinking, Willing and Feeling

2) Body, Soul and Spirit

In Christian teachings many are taught the concept of the Holy Trinity:

God - Son - Holy Spirit

In some metaphysical teachings it is expressed as:

Masculine, Feminine and Love

We are taught another trinity expression in psychology:

Conscious - Subconscious - Unconscious

The ancient mystics of Hawaii, the Kahunas, teach about our three levels:

Lower self - Middle self - Higher self

I feel a connection with three aspects of my being. I relate to this as my own personal trinity.

Conscious self (personality)

Higher Self (soul)

God Self (the God within me)

The awareness of this trinity within myself has helped me to connect with others who are experiencing their own personal trinities. Our relating is on a much deeper level when we know who we truly are inside.

To say " I am God ", is not to be disrespectful. It is an acknowledgement that God lives within me. A spark of God is inside of me. We are all children of God. It says in the Bible that we are " made in God's image ". I do not believe that God is an old man with a beard. Personally, I don't believe that God has a gender. God is an essence and a part of God's essence lives inside each one of us. Because God is within us, we are co-creators. We are co-creators with God, not without God.

When we awaken to the fact that we are co-creators of the Universe, a new realization occurs. <u>We can manifest miracles in our lives!</u>

My healing work has taken on a whole new meaning in my life. When I make the Trinity link, the energy that floods through me is much more intense.

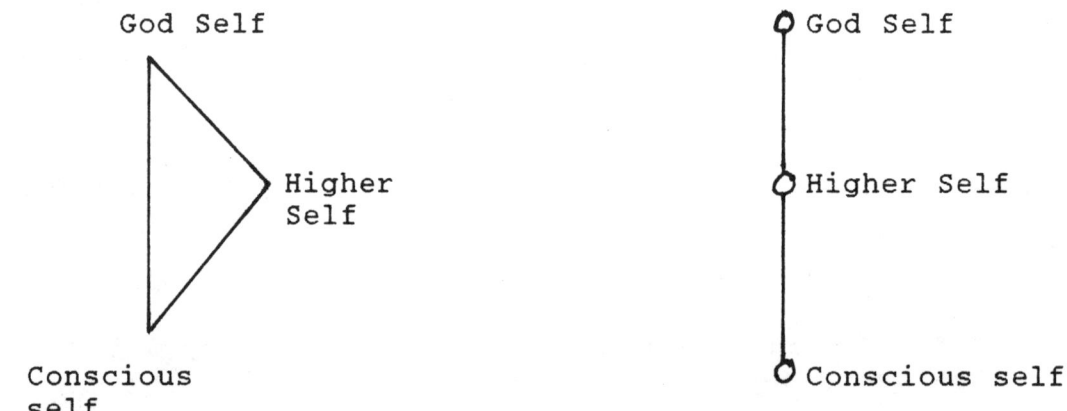

When I get relaxed and centered, then I become aware of my Higher Self connection. Once that connection has been made, I then raise my awareness and energy level to connect with my God Self. Each individual expression feels different and I am aware of that. The Higher Self feels less dense than my conscious self. The God Self feels lighter than the Higher Self level.

I have been channeling in my healing work on a conscious level for several years. I have taught many students how to channel the healing Love Light of the Universe. It was a natural step for me to go deeper within myself to a more advanced understanding of who I am. The personal trinity link-up has been a very powerful tool for my spiritual growth.

I have known for many years about all three aspects of my being. Many of us have known this. It is when you consciously connect with it and claim it as your truth that things begin to shift in your life. It is a higher level of commitment than what one may experience with only the Higher Self.

Make the connection and sense what you feel:

You are soul. What does that mean to you? Sense how it feels. (If you have not made this connection before, many of the techniques in this book will help you to do so.) Become one with your soul. You are soul. You are soul first. When your present life is over and you leave the physical plane, you will still be soul. You are soul.

God lives within you. A spark of God's Divine Essence is within you. Sense the spiritual flame in your heart center. Acknowledge your God Self. You are a part of God, therefore you are a God. You are a co-creator. You are a co-creator of the Universe. You are a creator of your own personal universe. Wherever you go, you take your universe with you.

You are responsible for your own life. You are responsible for your own happiness. You are you. You are soul. You are God. You are you.

Trinity   Link-Up   Process

Conscious awareness of:

your Conscious self (personality)

your Higher Self (soul)

your God Self (the God within you)

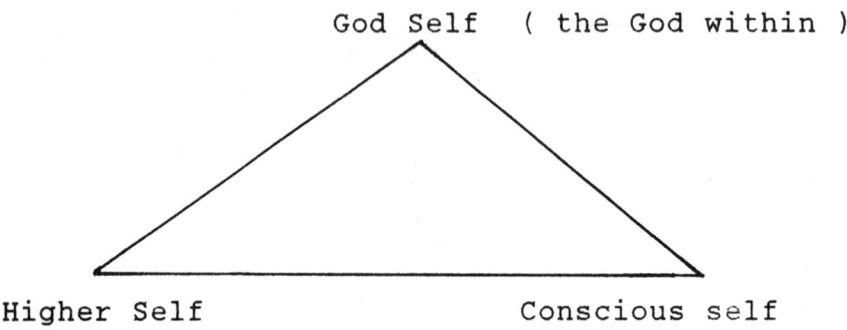

When you consciously connect with these three parts of
yourself, you will raise your awareness level. Once you
acknowledge your union with your Higher Self and the God within
you, all things become possible.

You are not being disrespectful in saying, " I am God. "
You are just acknowledging that a part of God's essence is inside
of you.

Trinity Link-Up Process and More

Be in a relaxed state.

Be aware of how your body feels.

Be aware of how dense it feels.

Allow yourself to relax more. Take some slow, deep breaths.
Feel your body relaxing and getting lighter.

Feel yourself expanding as you get lighter.

Consciously connect with your Higher Self. Feel how light the
sensation is.

After you have made the connection with your Higher Self, allow
yourself to expand even more. You will feel a new level of
lightness. You will feel a higher level that you are connecting
with as you become lighter.

Consciously connect with your God Self. Feel how much lighter the
sensation is compared to how you felt with the Higher Self
connection. It is a lighter sensation. There is a feeling of
more expansion.

When you have connected with the God within you, your God Self,
then you are ready to go to a higher level. You are ready to
connect your personal universe with that of the Great Universe.

Allow your energies to expand outward. Become one with yourself
and one with the Universe. You feel one with everything and
everyone. You feel one with the Universe. You feel no
separation. You feel a blending taking place. You are in
communion with your energies and with the energies of God. This
is the feeling that many of the great mystic saints have written.
You are sharing in their experience NOW!

MY PERSONAL EXPERIENCE:

HEALING

HEALING   DO'S   and   DON'TS

Be in a calm, relaxed state.

Center and focus your attention on your client.

Be here and now. Be there for your client. Don't be thinking of
other things, other people.

Be attentive to your client's needs. If your client is getting
in touch with emotional issues and crying, give him or her a
tissue. If your client looks cold and is shaking, cover her or
him with a blanket.

Be in touch with any inner messages that you get whether they be
visions, associations of similar situations, words, or other
thoughts. You may feel guided to share these with your client
later. You may choose to share these and you may take them into
your next meditation practice for future and deeper understanding.

Be open to the experience, the other person and yourself. The
more open you are, the more you will channel healing energy
through you.

When you begin to channel healing energy through you, always fill
up your heart and take for yourself first. The more you love
yourself, the more you will love others, the more you can give to
others.

If it is permissible in your working environment, light a candle.
The candle is the focal point into which you and your client may
release any negative energy.

At the end of the session, ground your energy. Some practitioners
wash their hands, others just shake off excessive energy, while
others place their hands on the floor or ground to release the
energy.

After the session is over you will need to spiritually cleanse the
room. This can be done between sessions or at the end of the day.
You can spiritually cleanse a room in many ways.

    1) with the mind, you can project the intention that your
working space is cleared of any negative energy.

    2) in addition to this, you can use a candle or burn sage and
cedar and smudge the space.

HEALING   NO-NO'S

Don't ever offer to do a healing on someone. You can let others know that you have a healing practice, but don't push yourself on others. This involves an ego issue for many people. If it is some one in your immediate family, then that is a different situation. You are already involved. If people truly want you to do a healing session with them, then they will come to you.

Don't ever do a healing when you are sick or exhausted.

Don't ever do a healing when there is alcohol or non-prescription drugs in your body.

Don't ever do a healing on a client who has alcohol or non-prescription drugs in his / her body.

Don't ever claim that you can cure some one. God does the curing. You are only a vessel for the energy to pass through. You are an instrument of healing. It is not your energy, but God's energy that helps others.

Don't be attached to the results of a healing session. If you do and the client doesn't get better, then you will blame yourself. Some people are not meant to get better. It is part of their spiritual plan. If your clients do get better and you are attached to this, then you will end up being egotistical. There is no room for ego in healing work. You are in service to others. Be humble and appreciative that the Universe has supported you.

Don't ever diagnose a client. Don't ever prescribe anything for a client. These actions place you at the risk of practicing without a license. Some states have been known to enforce this action by placing practitioners in jail!

Some practitioners in healing work are aware of working with the energies of their spirit guides. This can be a wonderful experience, but it can dampen if you become boastful about the entities you channel. I see this occurring more and more frequently with the phenomena of channeling. Like anything else, the more a person brags, the more insecure he / she really is inside. The more one brags, the more ego is involved. The more there is ego, the less clear the channel. To have Light, there is no room for ego. Just love yourself. Just be yourself.

110

A Prayer for Healing

Divine Creator: Father, Mother, Son as One: We open ourselves up
fully to receive the Healing Love Light of the Universe. It is
our birthright to receive this Divine Light and we are truly
worthy to receive this Divine Essence. We surround, fill and
protect ourselves with this Healing Light. We ask for a blessing
of our unity as our energies come into communion with each other
and with those energies of the Universe. We are open to all
healing that is to take place on all levels of our being. It is
good. It is done. So be it.

Prayer of Protection

The Light of God surrounds us.

The Love of God enfolds us.

The power of God protects us.

The presence of God watches over us.

Where ever we are, God is.

1.

1. Used by permission of Dr. Frank Alper, Arizona Metaphysical
Society, Phoenix, Az.

These are powerful affirmations. Say each one slowly until you
have fully absorbed the meaning and energy of the statement.

Affirm out loud:

I have peace.

I channel peace.

I am peace.

I am open to love.

I channel love.

I am love.

I am surrounded and filled with Light.

I channel Light.

I am Light.

I am surrounded with healing energy.

I channel healing energy.

I am healing energy.

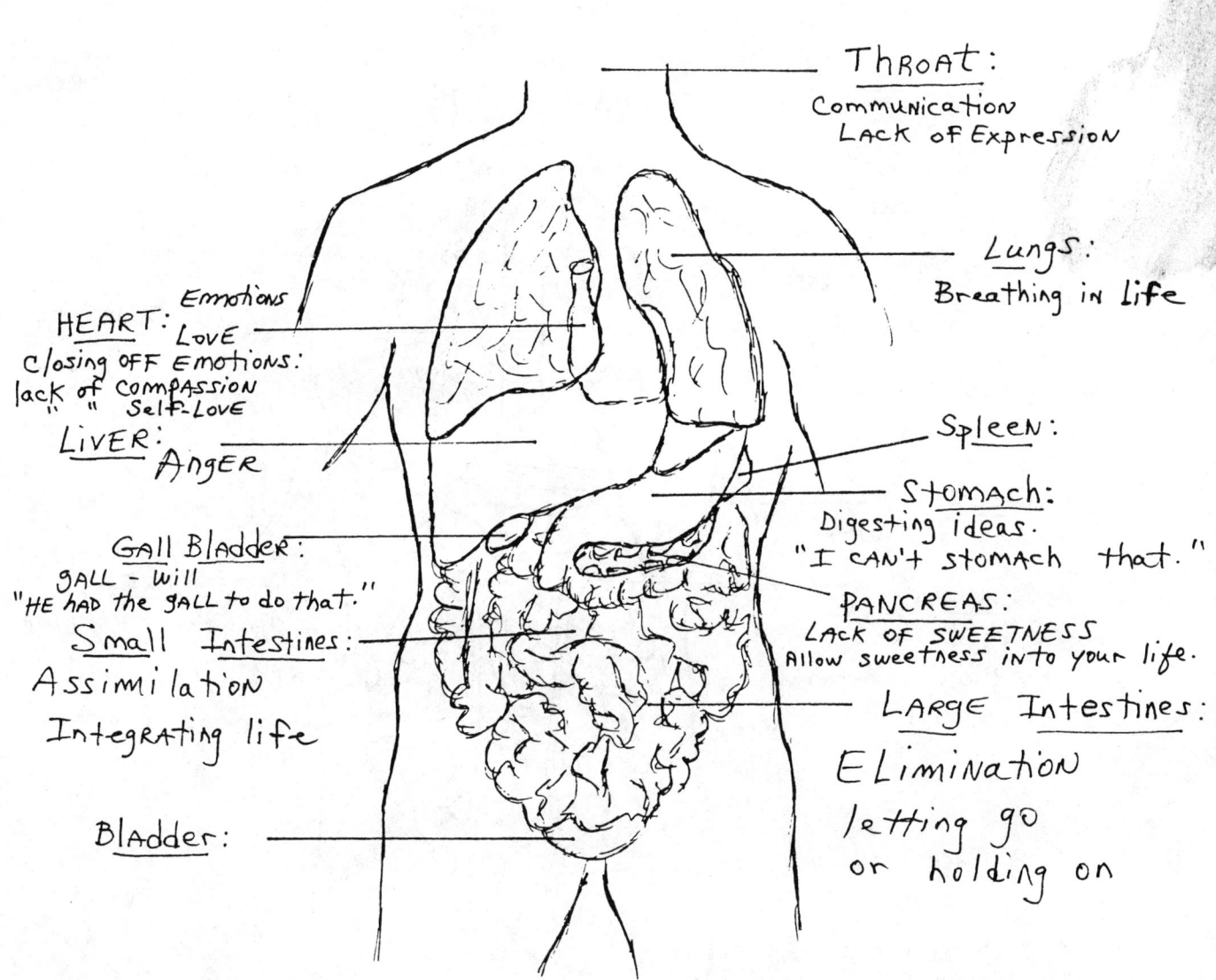

THROAT:
Communication
Lack of Expression

Lungs:
Breathing in Life

HEART: Emotions
LOVE
Closing OFF Emotions:
lack of Compassion
"   "   Self-Love

LIVER:
Anger

Spleen:

Stomach:
Digesting ideas.
"I CAN't stomach that."

GALL Bladder:
gALL - Will
"HE HAD the gALL to do that."

PANCREAS:
LACK of SWEETNESS
Allow sweetness into your life.

Small Intestines:
Assimilation
Integrating life

LARGE Intestines:
ELimiNation
letting go
or holding on

Bladder:

F R O N T

113

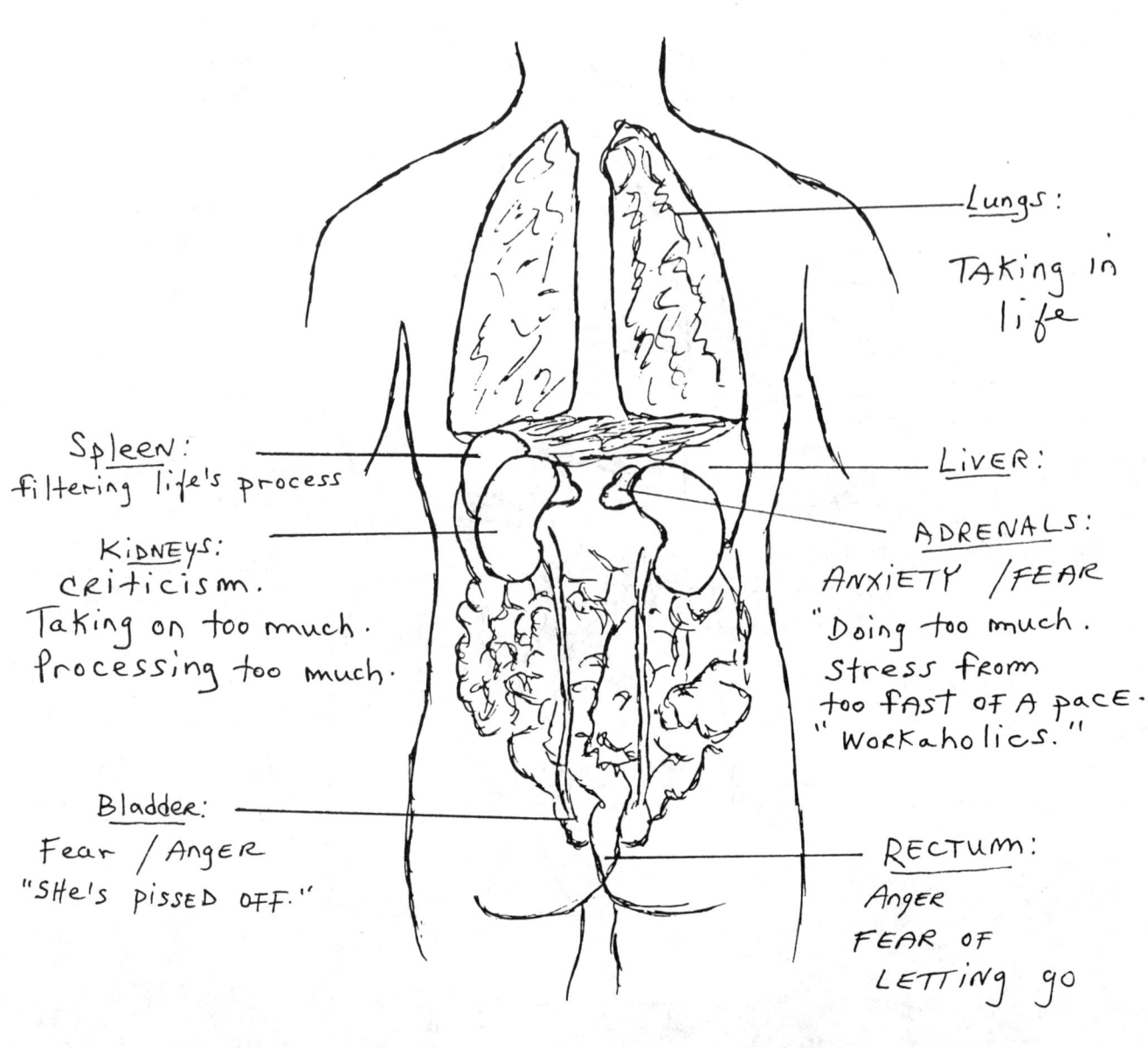

Lungs:
Taking in life

Spleen:
filtering life's process

Liver:

Kidneys:
Criticism.
Taking on too much.
Processing too much.

Adrenals:
Anxiety /Fear
"Doing too much.
Stress from
too fast of a pace.
"Workaholics."

Bladder:
Fear / Anger
"She's pissed off."

Rectum:
Anger
Fear of
Letting go

B A C K

How to Measure Energy Imbalances

You can locate energy imbalances by measuring the chakra centers. This is described in my book, <u>Crystal Therapeutics</u> on pages 84 through 86. Another way to locate imbalances is to finger test. You can use a pendulum. The client holds his / her hand open. You can place the pendulum directly over the energy points. See the two finger charts on the following pages. If the pendulum goes clockwise, then that area checks out okay. If it goes counter clockwise, then there is an imbalance in that area. You can also do this technique on yourself. You can have one hand open, while the other hand holds the pendulum and measures the area. It is your intention that counts. You can ask, " What is the energy in this area? " Or you can ask, " Is this area in balance? " Hold the pendulum over the area and see which direction it rotates.

Another way to measure these areas is with the technique known as Applied Kinesiology, or muscle testing. You can measure your client's hand in the following manner:

The client extends an arm out. Tell the client to hold it there. Gently push down at the forearm area, until the arm locks into place. Feel where it locks. That gives you a feel as to how the client's muscles test. That is known as " testing in the clear. "

Next, you can test each energy point of the client's hand. Have the client use his / her thumb to point to the energy points in the same hand. For example: To test the small finger, the client can hold the thumb and small finger together to form an " O ". This completes a circuit of energy. To test the ring finger, the client can hold the thumb and ring finger together at the tips. To test the middle finger, the thumb and middle finger are connected at the tips. To test the index finger, the thumb and index finger are held at the tips. To test the thumb, the thumb is held at the other end of the same hand, below the small finger.

The finger test is done in one hand, while the other arm is muscle tested. Both actions are done together at the same time, to be an effective test. For example: I want to check out a client's emotional state. I can have the client hold out an arm for me to muscle test. At the same time, he / she has taken the thumb and ring finger (of the hand opposite the arm being tested) and connects them together. If the arm does not lock into place, while the fingers in the opposite hand are being tested, then there is an imbalance on an emotional level. I can then muscle test to see what therapies would be appropriate and a priority. This is a good idea if you are trained in several healing modalities.

I would then muscle test an arm to check out what therapy is a priority: MariEl healing, flower essence counseling, Reiki Healing, regression work, Rebirthing, or any other emotional healing technique. If the arm locked on one, more than the other methods tested, then that would be the technique that I would choose. I use crystals in many of the various healing modalities that I have been trained in for my session work.

Other pointers with finger testing: I recommend the book, The Science and Art of the Pendulum by Gabriele Blackburn for pendulum work.

You can also ask for the order of priorities in therapy work and areas of imbalance. Many clients may have the emotional and etheric points out of balance. Which one is more balanced than the other? Which one needs more healing? If you are clear with your questions when you are asking for guidance, then your answers will be more clear.

You can use the open hand to test. I do this for measuring the multiple bodies of a client. A pendulum can be held over the open hand of the client, or yourself. Ask, " What is the energy level of the physical body? " " What is the energy of the etheric body? " Do the same for the lower and higher mental bodies, causal body and spiritual body. If the different bodies are out of balance, the pendulum will rotate counter clockwise. The rotation occurs, while the pendulum is held over the palm chakra and that particular body is being mentioned. I usually do this in silence to myself. Most of the clients whom I measured a few years ago, had a point of balance and imbalance. It usually occurred around the lower and higher mental bodies or the higher mental body to the causal body. I would measure before the healing session and then recheck it after the session work was completed.

Another energy diagnostic tool is to use dowsing rods, such as the Cameron Aurameter or the " L rods ". They can be used to measure the energy field of the clients before and after the session work. It is good for the clients to witness this measurement for themselves.

All of these techniques are tools for growth. I used them at the beginning of my practice. They helped to open me to explore my inner guidance system. I now no longer need them, but feel that they are worth mentioning to other healing practitioners who may not have experimented with them.

All of the energy measurement information is written down in my session sheets. It is recorded and kept for future use. If a client returns for more than one balancing session, it is nice to have a comparison of the patient's progress. I have included a few different session sheets in my book, Crystal Therapeutics. They are available to those who have a healing practice. You can purchase my book at your local bookstore, or write to the Holistic Health Works.

I learned from my ambulance days how important it is to keep records of everything. You never know when a documented statement will come in handy. It is also important to take a medical history of every new patient. I once had a client go into a grand mal seizure in front of me. He had forgotten to take his medication. I would have been more prepared, if I had known that he was epileptic and on a prescribed medication.

A final note: I highly recommend that you take training in First Aid and CPR. What if you are alone with your client and an emergency arises? What are you going to do? How are you going to handle the situation? You are in service work. You owe it to your clients as a professional to be trained in these basic, but important techniques. Call your local chapters of the American Red Cross and the American Heart Association.

ENERGY DISTORTION POINTS IN HAND

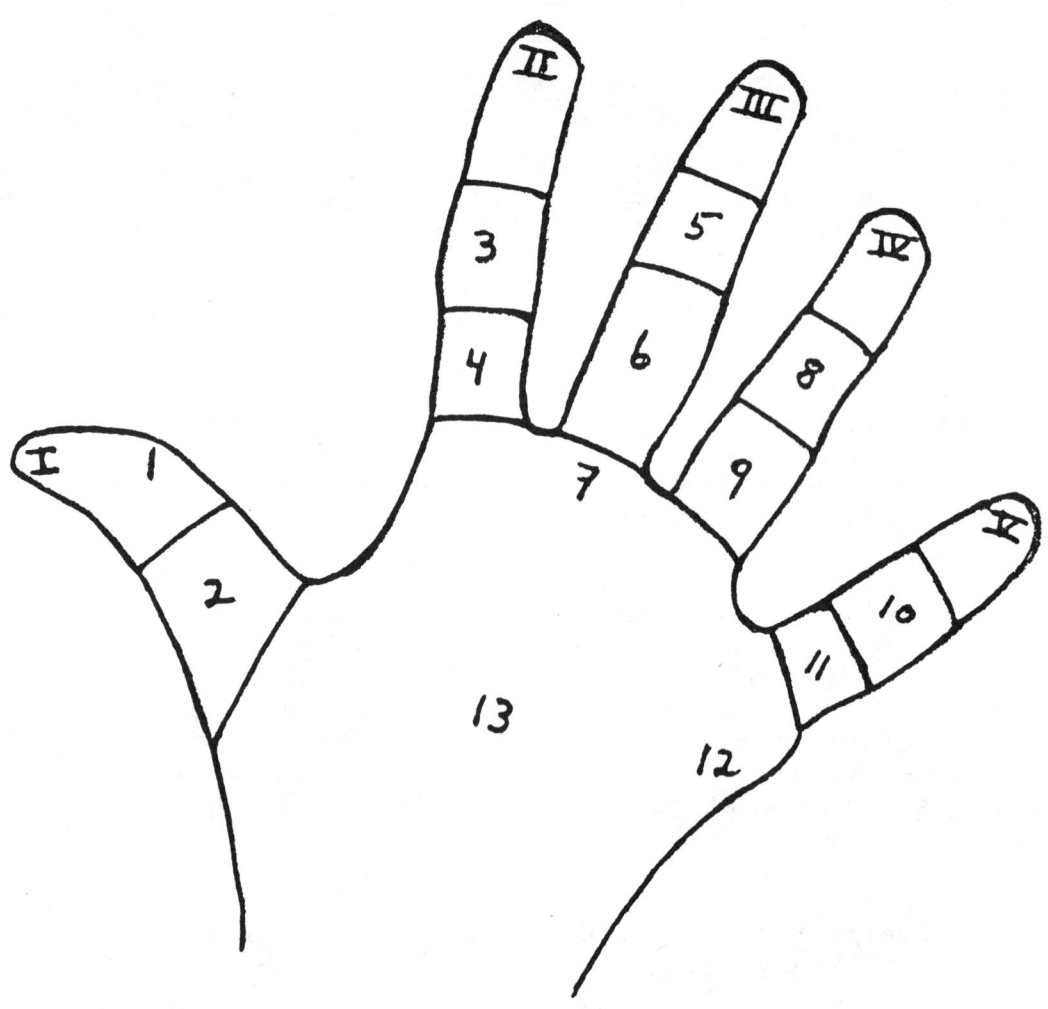

I	NERVOUS SYSTEM — Brain — Physical Energy
	1 Etheric Energy
	2 Acid Alkali Balance
II	RESPIRATORY SYSTEM
	3 Bronchial
	4 Lungs
III	DIGESTIVE SYSTEM
	5 Liver
	6 Stomach
	7 Intestines
IV	URINARY SYSTEM
	8 Kidneys
	9 Bladder
V	REPRODUCTIVE SYSTEM
	10 Male: Testes — Prostate
	Female: Uterus — Ovaries
	11 Genitals
12	BLOOD CONDITION & CIRCULATION
13	HEART FUNCTION

FROM THE SCIENCE AND ART OF THE PENDULUM
By permission of Idylwild Books
© COPYRIGHT GABRIELE BLACKBURN 1983

ENERGY POINTS and RELATED HEALING THERAPIES

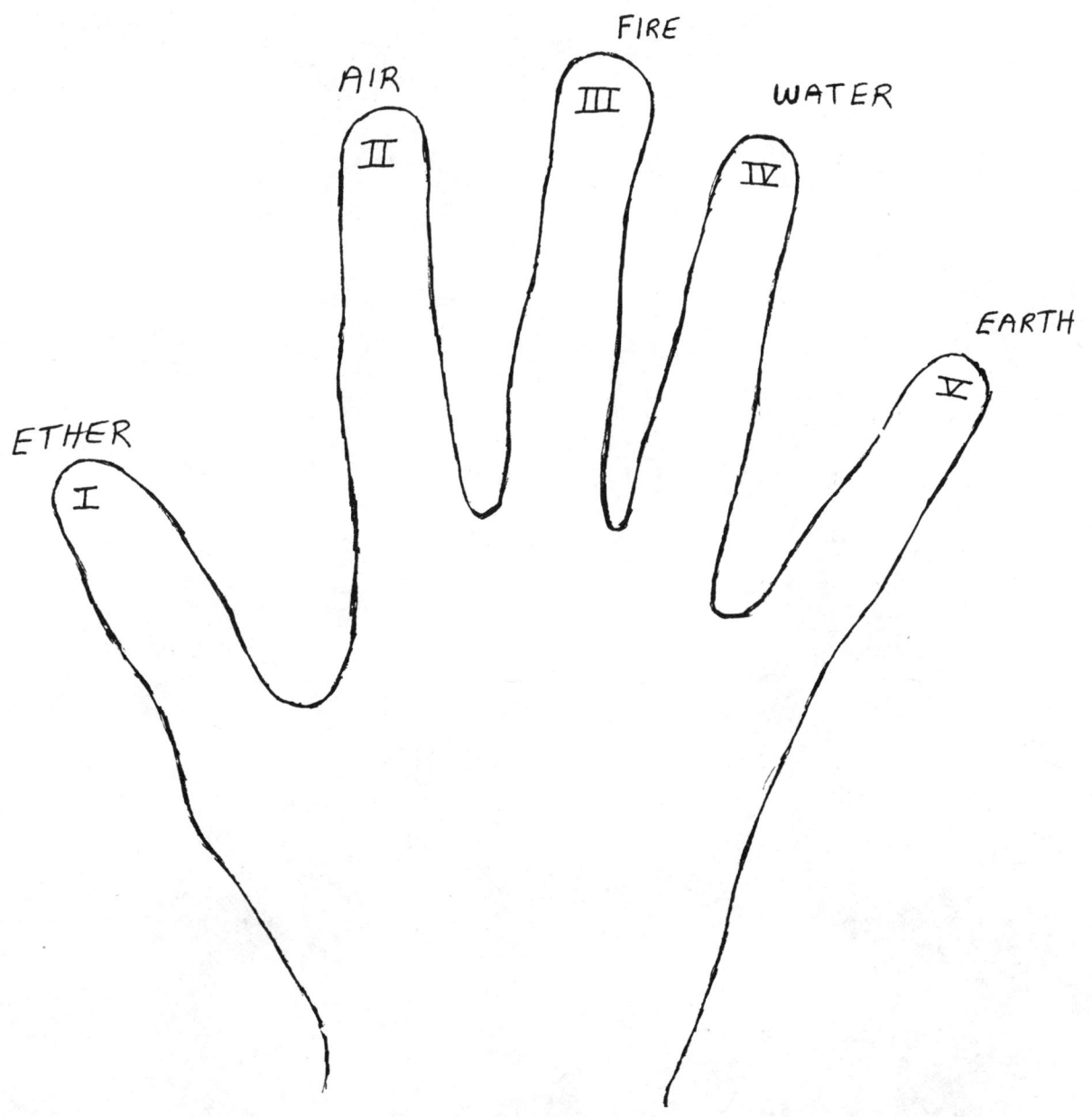

Techniques To Balance Areas:

I- Soul Work: Etheric (Chakra Balancing), Shantira Chakra Therapy, Color Healing Therapies

II- Breathing: Yoga Breathing, Color Breathing, Polarity work with Breath (Wayne Cook Technique)

III- Digestion: Dehydration, Diet, Colonic Irrigation, Fasting

IV- Emotional: ESR, Flower Essence Counseling, MariEl Healing, Reiki Healing, Regressions, Rebirthing

V- Physical: TFH, Massage Work, Meridian Balancing, Jin Shin Do, Shiatsu, Polarity Therapy, Reiki Healing

CRYSTAL   HEALING   MEDITATIONS

Pre-meditation   Technique

This technique is good to do for those who have trouble relaxing and emptying their minds. It came to me one Sunday at the London Grove Quaker Meeting. Even if you are an advanced meditator, there may come times when you need to get out of your mental process. I hope this technique helps you, as it has helped me on occasions.

Close your eyes and take some slow, deep breaths. Allow your body to relax.

See yourself entering a room. Go through the doorway. You notice on your right that there is a corner closet. Go over to the closet and unlock the door. As you open it, you see that inside the closet there are a few shelves. Take some deep breaths. Remove from your mind anything that is bothering you. Remove any distracting ideas, thoughts or feelings that you've been carrying around with you. Place them on the shelves.

One by one, you put them away on the shelf. Release any anxieties and place them on the shelf. Release any fears and place them on the shelf. Release any thoughts or feelings that make you uncomfortable and place them on another shelf. Piece by piece, you are unloading your mind. As you do this, you feel lighter inside. It helps you to become more relaxed. You begin to feel peace inside of yourself. Continue placing any thoughts and feelings that surface onto the shelves. (Pause for three to five minutes.)

When you feel empty and clear from this releasing process, close the door. Lock the door with the key. Put the key in your pocket. Remember that all of those thoughts and feelings are in the closet. You can collect them later, if you choose.

Turn around and go over to the meditation altar. Sit down in front of the altar and begin your meditation session. Take some slow, deep breaths. Open the top of your head (crown chakra) and allow the healing Light of the Universe to enter into your being. Direct this healing energy throughout your whole body. Ground the energy through your feet and down into the earth. You are now in balance to continue your meditation. Be at peace with yourself, for that is what you are.

CRYSTAL HEALING MEDITATION for EXHAUSTION

Pre-cleanse.

Smudge yourself.

Spiritual Cleansing Bath: 1 cup of sea salt, 1 - 2 cups of apple cider vinegar. Fill up the tub with warm water and add the two ingredients. (No crystals are needed for this bath.)

Immerse yourself fully three times. (Move your body in different positions to completely cover it with the bath water.) Fifteen minutes is the minimum time for this bath.

Crystal   Work

Supplies needed: three palm size, clear quartz crystals and one clear quartz cluster.

Collect all of the supplies and place them on your abdomen.

Lie flat on your back. You can use the floor, your bed or a healing table.

Place one crystal at your throat area with the point directed towards your chest.

Place the cluster over your thymus area (located between the throat and heart area).

Place the remaining two crystals in each hand. The points should be both directed towards your shoulders. You have created a triangle. The focal point is the thymus area.

Rest in this position for fifteen minutes. Visualize your energy being in perfect balance. See yourself whole, well and perfect. Be in touch with your energy. Sense how it feels.

When you are done, slowly sit up. You may feel very lightheaded and will need to remain seated for a few minutes to adjust to your new energy level. You can ground* yourself to speed up this process.

* This technique is further described in Crystal Therapeutics.

MY PERSONAL EXPERIENCE:

Harmonic Convergence Crystal Bath

Supplies:

Four crystals in each corner of the tub frame pointing inward to the center.

Two palm size crystals.

One crystal at your feet. (Point of the crystal is aimed away from your body.)

Four discharging crystals are lined up in front of you and are ready for use.

* *

Take one discharging crystal in both hands and place the crystal point away from you. Hold the crystal over the second chakra in your lower abdominal area. Exhale and breathe into the crystal. Release all blockages from the chakra area. As you do this, slowly move the crystal away from the body. Do this until you feel complete with releasing in that area. Remove the crystal and place it outside the bath area.

Take another discharging crystal and repeat the same procedure over the solar plexus area.

Repeat the same process over the heart center.

Repeat the same process over the throat center.

Complete this exercise with holding the two palm crystals:

The left hand crystal is pointing up towards the shoulder. The right hand crystal is pointing down and away from the body. When you feel guided, take the left hand with the crystal and touch it to the crown chakra. The right hand with the crystal is held at the root chakra. The left hand moves down to the brow with the crystal point aimed at the forehead area. Continue to move the left hand with the crystal down to the throat, heart, solar plexus and navel chakra. On completion of this exercise, both hands and crystals meet each other at the root chakra area. Visualize grounding your energies into the earth. Feel yourself rooted into Mother Earth.

MY PERSONAL EXPERIENCE:

Healing Tepee Meditation

Lie down. Take some slow, deep breaths and allow your body to relax.

Close your eyes and allow your body to relax on a deeper level.

Visualize a meadow. See yourself standing out in the meadow. As you look out into the distance, you see an Indian village. You are drawn to the direction of the village. You begin to walk towards the village. (Pause for two minutes.)

You have arrived at the Indian village. There are some children happily playing with a stick and stones. A few Native American women come over to you to greet you. You are welcomed here. You have come home.

The women take you to meet a medicine woman. You are taken to her tepee. She greets you and invites you into her healing space. This is a sacred sanctuary. Many healings have taken place here. You can feel the presence of all of those energies.

As a healer, you have shared so much of yourself with others. It is time for you to be the one receiving a healing session. You go over to the prayer blanket and lie on top of it. You begin to relax and open up to the healing energies of this sacred space.

The medicine woman anoints you with a healing oil. She chants a beautiful chant to bless you and her healing work. You are smudged with sage and cedar. She spiritually cleanses your energy field. You relax and deepen even more.

One by one, healing guides enter the tepee, a medicine man, an angel, a monk and a saint. They all surround you and begin to balance and heal you. You are open to this healing. You are open to their sharing and channeling the healing energy of the Universe. Take in this healing Light, now. Allow it to be received on all levels of your being. Bathe in this healing Light. You feel an energy connection with all of your healing guides. You are at peace with yourself. (Pause for five to ten minutes.)

The healing is complete now. You thank your healing guides for sharing their energies. You know you will meet each other again, from time to time. One by one, they leave the healing chamber. (Pause for two minutes.)

You are alone with the medicine woman again. You sit up and thank her for her sharing her healing space. She smiles and shares some teachings with you. She shares spiritual wisdom with you. Be open to the lessons shared. (Pause for three to five minutes.)

You are thankful for the teachings that the medicine woman shared with you. You embrace her and share energies together. She gently places her hand on your heart and sends healing energies to your heart center. You can feel your energy gently being raised. You are initiated by Spirit. Feel new energies awakening inside of you. You are ready to receive this on all levels of your being. (Pause for two minutes.)

The exchange is complete. You thank the medicine woman once more and leave her tepee. Outside, it is a brand new day. You are seeing it with a whole, new perspective. You are <u>really</u> seeing it. You leave the village smiling to yourself. You know that you can return to this sacred place at any time. You will return here again and again and again. This is one of your many homes. This is you.

Slowly bring your awareness back to this room and moment. Allow your body to stretch out. Awaken now. You are fully awake.

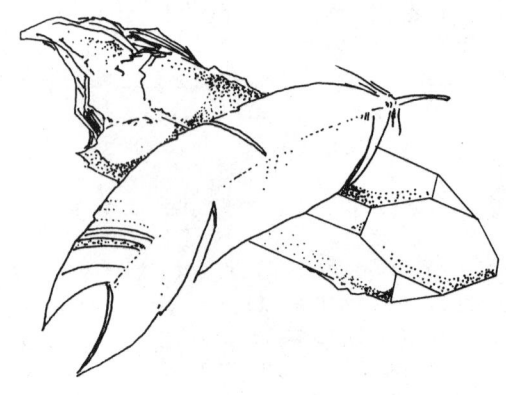

MY PERSONAL EXPERIENCE:

HEART   CLEARING

You will need two crystals for this exercise. One is for removal of the invisible fortress around your heart.

Take the crystal and go counter clockwise around the physical heart area to clear it. Once that process feels complete, remove the crystal and do the following:

Take another crystal and hold it between your palms. Project loving, healing thoughts into the crystal. (Pause for two minutes.)

Take the crystal and place it over the physical heart area. Sense the healing love vibration going into the heart area.
(Pause for five minutes.)

Take the crystal and place it at the center of your mid chest. Feel the heart chakra area balancing out.

Bathe in the healing Love Light of the Universe. You are truly worthy to receive this love. Feel your heart expanding and becoming lighter. The heaviness has been released. You are filled now with healing Light. Be one with the Light.

Warning: Do not do this exercise with quartz if you have a heart condition. You can clear the area with the healing energy of your palm chakras that you channel through you. If you have a pacemaker, do not ever put quartz in your energy field.

MY   PERSONAL   EXPERIENCE:

Inner Cave Meditation

Get in a relaxed position.

Do a breathing technique. You can take some slow, deep breaths,
or you may choose to do another advanced breath technique of your
choice.

Breathe normal and quiet the mind. The body feels very relaxed.

You can activate your brow chakra by focusing on it. As the mind

is blank, it looks into a dark cave. You go inside the cave.

There are no lights. There is only the light from outside the

entrance of the cave. It takes a lot of courage to walk into this

dark cave. You do not know what lies ahead of you. As you walk

into the cave, you slowly begin to lose the light behind you. It

becomes darker in front of you with each step that you take. You

go to one of the sides of the cave, so that you can sense where

you are walking. You may choose to walk down the center of the

path. You stretch your hands out in front of you. With each

courageous step that you take, you walk farther and deeper into

the cave. There is only you and the cave. There is only you and

darkness. You continue to journey inward. It is a long journey

into darkness. You have the courage to take this journey.

Everything you have done before this moment has been a preparation

for now. Continue to go farther into the darkness. You are alone

in the darkness.

With every step that you take and the farther you journey inward, the more you will be rewarded. Your knowing this is what gives you the initiative to go farther inward. The cave is like a maze. It curves to the left and to the right. You keep feeling your way forward with each step that you take. You come to another bend; you secure your footing and you go around the bend. As you go around the bend, you see a small glimmer of light. You go over to the light source. It is a magic crystal. You pick up the crystal in your hands. The small crystal sheds a little light on where you are and where you are headed. You continue along the path. The crystal light helps you to see for a while. As a few moments go by, the light of the crystal slowly grows dim. You are alone again in the darkness. You choose to continue to go along the path. The inward journey into this cave is also an inward journey into yourself. This is why you are here. You are here to grow, to explore, to journey. You continue along the path in darkness and alone. You are not afraid. You feel secure within yourself. You are a little anxious about the unfamiliar things that lie ahead, but you are strong within yourself. You come to another bend and you gently take the turn around the bend. In the distance is a light. It is the light of another light crystal. It shines more brightly than the first one. You go over and pick it up. It guides you along your path. The light is brighter.

As you walk with this light, the light glows twice as long in length of time than the last crystal light. You have gone much deeper into the cave. Slowly, the light of the second crystal goes out. You place the crystal in your pocket along with the other crystal. You do not discard the crystals. When you are done with your journey, you can place these crystals in the rays of the sun. The sun will charge them and they each will gain their light again. Continue your journey and go deeper into the cave. There are several bends in the path in front of you. Each time you go around a bend, there is a light that you know is ahead in the distance. As you walk closer to it, it becomes brighter. The source of the light is not in view, but you are slowly walking into the light. Around another bend, your path becomes clearer and there is more light. As you go towards the light, you now begin to see clearly in front of you with each step that you take. You go around one more bend and ahead of you is the source of the light. It is a large space of brilliant light. On the ground in front of you are crystals, jewels and treasure chests. You walk over to this chamber of crystal lights. You are curious about what lies inside of each treasure chest. You see a treasure chest and you walk over to it. You open up the chest and inside is a golden light. Inside are many scrolls, many teachings. This is the chest of spiritual wisdom. You can read from any of these paper scrolls anything that you choose to learn.

Many of the questions that you've carried around inside of you throughout your life can now be answered. Reach in and find a teaching that explains the answers you have been searching for. Reach inside now for an answer to a question, or several questions that you have had inside of yourself. You know which ones you would like to have answered now. This is your gift of all-knowingness. It is your time to explore this great opportunity. All of the answers that you ever seek are inside of you. It is your time to have your many questions answered. You may do so now.

(Pause for five to ten minutes.)

It is time now to leave this space. You can take some of the scrolls with you. You leave some of the others. You close the treasure chest for now. Some of the other treasure chests at this time are locked. You know that at another time when you journey inward within yourself, you will have an opportunity to grow even more. You know inside that another treasure chest will be opened up for you on your next journey. You will come back to this space again to learn the answers to your many questions. You will experience the true understandings to many situations in your life. This is your sanctuary. This is your wisdom sanctuary. You take a lighted crystal cluster that shines brightly. You have the scrolls, your papers with the teachings and you have the crystal cluster of light.

You are thankful for this experience and you now walk away with the light behind you. You are wiser now than when you entered the cave. Some questions have been answered. Understandings have been acknowledged. As you walk down through the winding turns of the cave, you see clearly. As you journey outward, the crystal lights of the cluster shine your way. You are no longer in darkness and you walk outside the mouth of the cave. The cluster is still lit and you place it on the ground. You take the two crystals in your pocket and place them on the ground also. The cosmic rays of the sun charge the crystals. You have these lights now. The next time that you journey inward to the cave, you have the crystal lights to guide your path. These crystal lights represent wisdom. Once you have learned, understood and acknowledged, then you can not return to a place of ignorance that you may have once experienced. You have raised your awareness. You have raised your consciousness. You have raised your understanding. Each time that you return, you will be wiser than the time before. You will have more light with you when you walk the path of the cave and journey inward. Each time that you seek an answer, it is within. You can return to this space, this wisdom sanctuary of your inner self at any time. It is yours to explore, if you choose to do so.

There is peace within yourself for having taken the courage to journey through darkness to find the light. You have been rewarded. Each time that you go into the cave, there are more jewels and more rewards for your efforts. The storehouse is unlimited. The supply is endless. You may notice from time to time as you journey inward that there seem to be new treasure chests that were not there before. As you raise your awareness and your vibration, you reach a higher level of perception. Each time you will perceive more clearly. You will sometimes see things that were not there before. They were there before; you just had not reached a level of seeing them. As you expand your awareness and your vision, you will see more around you. You will understand things more clearly on many levels. Congratulations for taking the journey inward.

Blessings be with you and may you always walk the path of Light.

Omalya

(This meditation was channeled while holding an elestial crystal cluster.)

MY PERSONAL EXPERIENCE:

POTPOURRI

CRYSTALS & DREAMING

How to start remembering your dreams:

Supplies: one notebook, black felt tip pen, and one quartz crystal.

Before going to bed, place a notebook and a pen next to your bed. Hold your crystal in your hands and program the intention: " This crystal will aid me in remembering my dreams. " Put the crystal under your pillow, or wear a small pouch with a neck chain and place the crystal inside the pouch. As long as the crystal is in your energy field, it will affect you.

One of your last thoughts prior to sleeping should be to ask your spirit guide to aid and protect you while you sleep. Ask to remember your dreams.

As soon as you wake up in the morning, reach over and grab your pen and notebook. Write down your thoughts. (The felt tip pen is good for this writing. It flows nicely without you having to focus a lot.) Write down some of the images you can recall from your dreams.

Later, when you get a chance, you can take your dream writing into your meditation to get a deeper understanding of what the dream was all about.

If you awaken by a clock, keep it close to your bed, so you can turn it off and then reach for the pen and notebook. Once you get out of bed, or share your dream with another person without writing it down, chances are that you will forget it completely.

You can learn a lot by keeping a dream journal. As you look back at a later date, you will have a clearer understanding of previous dreams. You also may notice one of them has actually taken place.

Other stones to dream with are: " Herkimer Diamond " quartz crystals, lapis lazuli, other blue stones, purple stones and white stones. These stones are for activation of the upper chakras. They are good for dreaming and meditation.

As you program yourself to remember your dreams and try some of the above suggestions, you will remember your dreams. Your remembering will go slowly at first; then it will become more consistent.

Crystals for Conception, Pregnancy and Birth

This vision came to me after having a dream. In the dream, I met a light being and we made love. This could represent many things in an awakened consciousness: a connection with my Higher Self, a connection with the Hierarchy or Heavenly Bodies, a connection with my spirit guide, or with a space being. Whatever the case may be, the pattern for using crystals came immediately to me as I began to awaken.

Crystal Pattern for Conception

Pre-cleanse: take a basic crystal bath (as described in my book, Crystal Therapeutics).

Gather the following supplies:
    - four candles
    - sage, cedar, sweetgrass and smudging supplies
    - eight chakra crystals, or small - medium size crystals
    - nine medium - large crystals (one should be a polished crystal)
    - ten to twenty large, palm size crystals (These will be used for the circle pattern.)

Locate a private, healing space.

Smudge the space with sage, cedar and sweetgrass.

Place a sheet or a blanket on the floor or ground surface.

Put the crystals in the center of your healing space.

Light a candle and place it in the East position of the space. Call in the Light forces of the East to protect and heal you. Feel a connection as you raise the candle out to the East and pull in those energies of Light. Repeat for the directions of the South, West and the North. Once you have connected with all Four Directions of sacred energies you can begin to lay out the crystals.

When making the circle pattern, your head will be pointing North and your feet are in the direction of the South.

Lie down on the floor and see how large your circle needs to be. Place the large crystals around you. Begin in the direction of the East, then place another crystal several inches away. Each placement of the crystal is in a clockwise direction (This follows the path of the sun.) Continue placing the large crystals around you until you have completed a circle.

Once you have the large crystals around you in a circle pattern, you are now ready to place the medium size crystals next. Place one at your feet, one in between your ankles, your calves, knees, thighs, hips and one polished crystal (it may be a small massage crystal point) at the genital area (on the ground in between your legs). All of these crystals are between your legs with the points aimed up toward your head. The seven medium size crystals are for channeling the Light energy.

Place the remaining two medium size crystals near where your hands will rest. You will use them later.

Place the eight small – medium size crystals (chakra crystals) on your seven chakra centers: 1) root chakra (represented on top of the genital area), 2) below the navel, 3) solar plexus, 4) heart center, 5) throat, 6) brow center, 7) top of the head (crown center), 8) above the head representing the Transpersonal Point: 12" – 18" above the crown chakra.

The remaining two crystals at the hands are now ready to be held. The left hand crystal is pointed up toward the shoulder. The right hand crystal is pointed down and away from the body. This coincides with the normal flow pattern of your energy: in the left and out the right side.

Do a Prayer of Protection again, calling on the Healing Love Light of the Universe to surround, fill and protect you. State that you are open to accept Healing Light energy into your vessel, your being.

Begin to visualize Healing Light energies traveling around the circle clockwise three times for a connection in the crystal energy field. After you have made the completion of the third cycle of energy, begin to direct the Healing Light to the crystals at your feet, ankles and up your legs. Channel the Light energy to your genital area. Focus the energy here for several minutes. Be open to receive Motherhood and sense a commitment to that. Be open to being a vehicle for a child of Light to enter you at this time. You are connecting consciously on a spiritual level. When you feel complete on focusing on this area, then continue channeling the Light energy up to the other chakra centers. Do this slowly and feel the connection at each chakra center. You have connected the root chakra through the crown chakra. Now, make the connection from your crown chakra to the Transpersonal Point. You have now completed the connection of Earth to Heaven.

Focus on your Heart Chakra. Place both your hands there while holding the hand crystals. See a spark of Light growing inside. Feel Love growing inside your heart. See love expanding and pouring outward throughout your entire being. (Pause for five minutes.)

Keep your left hand on your heart and place your right hand on your second chakra (abdomen area, below the navel). Feel a connection between your heart center and your sexual chakra. Visualize a rainbow bridge being created between your heart and the sexual chakra. Allow healing energies to balance out these centers together. (Pause for several minutes.)

Once you feel complete with this exercise remove all of the crystals. Keep the polished crystal to use for future use. Do not cleanse the polished crystal in sea salt water. You can place it on an amethyst cluster or smudge it. You want to hold the energies that you channeled in the healing meditation for the following stages of the pregnancy. You will cleanse the other crystals and use them again for other purposes. The polished crystal will never be used again for anything else, but the pregnancy.

The polished crystal is next to be used for your love-making with your partner. The crystal contains the spiritual seed energies. You may feel guided to hold it, share it with your partner to hold, or just have it near the both of you while you are making love.

After you physically conceive, you can meditate daily with the polished crystal placed at, or near your abdomen area (with the point up). It can be a communication tool for talking to the soul of your developing baby. It's like a spiritual telephone. It will amplify your thoughts and energy.

This crystal can also be with you during labor and delivery.*

This crystal can also be given to your baby after birth. It can be placed in a sewn or crocheted pouch and hung in the baby's crib.

What a joyous gift, a crystal that has been exposed to the energies from spiritual conception, physical conception, pregnancy and birth to a new life.

* Some women also take along " Herkimer Diamond " quartz crystals for labor. It has helped some women with their contraction pains. They squeeze the crystal during contractions. There is more discussion about Herkimers in my first book.

MORE   CRYSTAL   STORIES

Since my first book was published, I have experienced a few situations that I feel are important to share with my readers and students. As I travel and teach workshops, I come across some amazing crystal stories. Here are some that I witnessed happening to others.

This is the greatest, disappearing crystal story I've ever heard: Last summer, my company had a product booth displayed at a festival. I met a young woman and her mother there. The woman was in her early twenties. Both of the women were interested in the crystals and jewelry that we had displayed. We spent a good amount of time talking with each other. I noticed that the young woman was wearing an amethyst pendant. I also was able to sense that her energies were somewhat hyperactive and scattered. I showed the woman a smoky quartz pendant, but she was not interested in it at the time. Time went by and I kept meeting this woman on several occasions.

Several weeks later, I connected with this young woman one last time. She said, " You'll never believe what happened to me this week. I went horseback riding and the horse I was with, ate my amethyst crystal! The neck chain is still intact, but the crystal is gone! " I told her that it sounded like there was a message in it for her somewhere. I laughed and said that maybe the horse needed to cleanse himself, since amethyst is a cleansing agent. In any case, the horse knew. It took this event for the woman to open and explore another mineral for herself to wear. I tuned into her energy before and after I gave her a smoky quartz pendant to wear. She ended up purchasing it. After three hours she came back wearing the pendant. Her energy was so grounded. It was the most balanced I had ever seen her. This is a perfect example of two statements: If you are not meant to have a crystal, you will be guided to give it away, or it will disappear. Also, the crystal chooses you.

* *

I have had the opportunity to tune in to a few more customers and help them to select appropriate minerals for their energies. Everyone is at a different level of consciousness. One mineral may be appropriate for one person and inappropriate for another person. Each mineral affects everyone differently. Some crystal teachers overlook this important fact. Here are two important stories relating to this lesson.

I gave a lecture in New Jersey last year. After the lecture, my company had a product table with various crystal items on it. I offered my services for consultation for those who wanted to recheck crystals that they were interested in purchasing. One woman, in her fifties or sixties asked for a consultation. I had never met this woman before. I had her sit in front of me without any crystal products. I tuned into her energy. She was interested in purchasing a clear quartz sphere for her meditations. I had her hold it and tuned in again to her energy. As I attuned to her energies, I began to get severe chest pains. I asked her if she had a heart condition. She said, " Yes. " It was obvious to me that I had sensed her energy and how it had responded to the clear quartz. It was not my energy, because I can sit with a large, clear quartz sphere for hours in meditation and there are no chest pains. I took away the clear quartz and gave her a rose quartz sphere to hold.

Again, I attuned to her energy. This time, I noticed that there was no chest pain. The clear quartz had amplified her heart condition. The rose quartz had helped to balance it. As most crystal practitioners know, rose quartz balances the heart chakra and aids emotional healing. It was not appropriate for this woman to work with clear quartz. Her energy cannot handle it, at this time.

****

We are constantly growing and evolving. We need to learn to go inside and listen to our inner guidance. Some minerals are okay for us to work with, while others are not. As we raise our consciousness, we raise our energies. As we raise our energies, we are able to work with some minerals that we previously could not work with before. It is an ongoing process. I do not agree with many of the New Age retailers who tell their customers that everyone should start out with a clear quartz crystal. The woman with the heart condition is a perfect example that proves this untrue. It is much safer to begin crystal work with rose quartz. It is a more gentle mineral.

WARNING:

It was stated in my book, <u>Crystal Therapeutics</u> that all quartz crystals and products should be kept away from any people with heart pacemakers. NO QUARTZ AROUND PACEMAKER PATIENTS!!!! There are only a handful of crystal teachers who are sharing this message, Dr. Frank Alper and myself among them. I've sat in other crystal workshops and have never heard this message shared.

The old pacemakers ran on batteries and magnets. The newer ones are made with silicon chips (quartz). They can be programmed for many different functions compared to the older type. Each pacemaker has a set rhythm to aid the heart in a steady rate of a heartbeat. <u>If you put quartz near the pacemaker it may alter the rhythm of the pacemaker</u>. It may alter the heartbeat of the patient. One of my friends, Regina Hugendubler is a Certified Critical Care Nurse. She agrees with the information on quartz and pacemakers. I also take this message seriously from my exposure to working with heart patients, as an ambulance attendant in Colorado.

Regina says that now, in modern times, a pacemaker patient can check and alter the rhythm of the pacemaker by holding the telephone to the pacemaker. An adapting device helps to send a signal from the patient's phone, to the other end of the phone connection that has a computer hook up. The computer sends a signal to the computer silicon chip of the pacemaker and adjusts the rhythm, if it is needed. I also inquired about pacemakers and quartz with a friend, Stephen Ruback, who has done some work with pacemakers. Different wave length signals alter the rhythms of pacemakers. Do you recall seeing signs in restaurants stating: " Microwave oven in use. " It is practical to use common sense with heart patients. Be careful with the crystals. It is always safe to just do " laying on of hands " healing for them.

148

Here's another interesting story about minerals:

I was selling crystals at a product booth last year. Two women from California came to look at our crystal jewelry. One lady was guiding her roommate in the selection. She noticed that we had a black obsidian pendant in stock. She told her friend to buy it because she needed protection. I gave the pendant to the woman to hold. She held it in her hand for a few minutes. When it came time to give it to me, she could not open her hand. Her hand had tightened around the pendant. This did not feel right to me. It was an obvious sign that the black obsidian was not appropriate for this woman's energy. Her roommate kept telling her to buy it.

I offered to tune in to this woman's energy. She was open to that. We faced each other and I sensed her energy, while she held different pendants. I had the woman think about the situations, in which she felt she needed protection. As she thought about the situation, I " fine tuned " to her energies. The pendant that registered the best energy level for the situation was a clear quartz pendant with a faceted pink tourmaline. The black obsidian did not feel right for whatever she was thinking about, while I was tuning in to her energy. She then shared what was going on in her life and why she felt she needed protection. Her father had recently died and she had been very close to him. Both she and her roommate had experienced visitations from her father from the spirit world. He would " hang around " their apartment and of course, that would bother them. He even followed them to the East Coast. Both felt that the black obsidian would help the situation.

After hearing the whole story, I again tuned in to the woman's energy. This time I thought about the woman and her deceased father. The clear quartz and pink tourmaline registered the best support for this particular situation. I shared that this woman needed to release her father in love and send him to the Light. The black obsidian did not feel like the right stone for this situation. I told the woman that she was focusing on fear, if she felt she needed the black obsidian. It wasn't exactly a poltergeist that was hanging around her playing fun and games. It was her deceased father. Either he was still emotionally attached to her, or she was still attached to her memories of him. If she let go of the fear and focused on loving him, his soul would be supported to find the Light that it needed.

The woman went inside herself to check her own true feelings about what I shared with her. She bought the clear quartz with the pink tourmaline, even though her roommate kept telling her to buy the black obsidian. She chose to love her father, not fear him.

* * * * * * * * * * * * * * * * * * *

Another lady came to my booth once. She was a jockey and rode horses in high jump races. She asked what would be a good stone for focus and relaxation. She wanted something that would help her to be in balance as she raced with other jockeys. I had the woman think about being on the horse, making the high jumps. As she visualized the race, I tuned into her and sensed topaz for her mental clarity and apache tear (black obsidian) for grounding. She needed to be clear about what was ahead of her as she saw the jumps coming up. She needed to be in tune with the energy of the horse. By doing this, she and the horse could synchronize and clear the high fences together. The golden topaz would balance the solar plexus and aid in decision making. It also is a playful stone. It would help the jockey to lighten up. The black obsidian would help to ground this woman's energy. She had too much energy in her head because she concentrated too much on making the jumps. The obsidian would help to bring down some of that energy throughout her body.

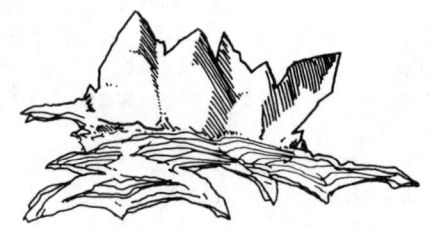

FIRST   AID   OIL

Arnica oil (Weleda), hypericum, calendula, rescue remedy, kunzite tinctures.

Safflower oil, almond oil; tinctures of: arnica, hypericum, calendula; flower essences: rescue remedy (Bach), self-heal (FES); and gem elixirs: kunzite, ruby and emerald.

Both of these formulas are great for: bruises, broken bones, (closed fracture), pulled ligaments, sprains, strains, and swelling.

The arnica is good for swollen areas. Use it on closed wounds and injuries. The hypericum is helpful for trauma involving nerve pain, such as crushed fingers. The flower, calendula is a soothing remedy used for cuts (unbroken skin), skin irritations and rashes.

The flower essences: Rescue Remedy is a combination of five of the Bach Flower remedies. It is excellent for shock or trauma to the body and mental process. Self-heal (FES) is a flower used for healing wounds and other imbalances.

The gemstone elixirs or tinctures: Kunzite contains lithium which balances the emotions. One of my crystal teachers, Fred Rubenfeld, gave me a piece to hold once. I placed it on a sore muscle. The pain went away within a short time. Ruby is good for circulating the blood flow. The red color balances blood disorders. Emerald is a master healer gemstone. It balances all of the meridians and chakras, especially the heart area. The color green is a master tonic for the body. It aids exhaustion.

For your oil base, you can use the above mentioned oils. My favorite massage oils are: Arnica Massage Oil by Weleda Products of Spring Valley, N.Y. and Aura Glow by Heritage Products in Virginia Beach, Va. The Aura Glow product is based on the Edgar Cayce readings. The Weleda oil is made from botanical products that are grown according to Rudolf Steiner's natural biodynamics method. You can write for a retail catalog from both Weleda and Heritage Products.

The homeopathic plant tinctures listed above can be ordered from: Boiron, 1208 Amosland Road, Norwood, Pa. 19074 (215) 532-2035. They carry an excellent homeopathic first aid kit and other products. Write for a retail catalog.

You are not the past.
You are the present.
You are now.

You are not the future.
You are the present.
You are now.

You are now.
You are now in this present moment.
You are now conscious in this present moment.
You are now aware in your present moment.

You are now.
You are light.
You are now feeling the light pouring through you.
You are becoming the light.
You are now the light.

You are now.
You are peace.
Feel the peace flowing through you
on all levels of your being.
Feel the peace quieting your mind.
Become one with the sensation of peace.
You are peace, now.

You are now.
You are love.
Feel love flowing through you.
Feel your heart expanding and blossoming with love.
Become one with the sensation of peace.
You are peace, now.
You are now.
You are love.
Feel love flowing through you.
Feel your heart expanding and blossoming with love.
Become one with the love vibration.
You are now.
You are love.

You are now.
You are truth.
You are truth expressed fully.
Truth flows through you in your actions,
in your thoughts and in your feelings.
You are now.
You are truth.

You are now.
You are compassion.
You are compassion shared with yourself
and with others.
You are now, compassion.

You are now.
You are purpose.
You are aware of your purpose.
You are aware that your purpose
will continue to evolve and change.
As you are aware, you will be purpose
in actions of light,
actions of truth,
and actions of love.

You are now.
Feel the present moment.
Feel the present moment blossoming and unfolding.
You are sensing the present moment fully.
You are experiencing your experience.
You have become one with your experience.
You are aware of the energy flowing through you.
You are totally aware of the sensations that you feel.
And you are aware of the thoughts
and feelings that you are experiencing.

You are one with your moment.

You are now.

SPIRITUAL   CLEANSING   and   RELEASING

Crystal Ceremony for Transformation

Supplies needed:

    - paper, pen and pad to write on
    - amethyst cluster, small or medium size
    - Burning Bowl (ceramic or metal)
    - sage, cedar, abalone shell and a feather
    - candle and wooden matches

Tear an 8 1/2 by 11" sheet of paper into four strips of equal size.

Place one on the note pad with a pen for immediate use. Put the other three paper strips aside for now. Place these to your left side.

Place the amethyst cluster to your left side.

Place the unlit candle and matches in front of you.

Place the burning bowl to your right side.

Prepare the sage and cedar in the abalone shell and place it unlit to your right side (to the right of the burning bowl).

Now, you are ready to begin.

<u>Relax and deepen</u>. When you feel relaxed and centered, upon your own cue begin the ceremony.

<u>Light the candle</u> in front of you. It represents the flame of life, the great Light of the Source, the Light within you.

Be quiet and reflect inward. (Pause.)

Think of one important issue that you would like to release at this time.

Write a simple sentence that expresses your desire to release this issue in your life.

Read this sentence of release three times. Pause in between each one and let your statement really sink into your mind. Be aware of what you choose to let go of at this moment in your life. (Pause.)

Fold the paper in half and then in half once again. Hold it above the candle flame. Allow yourself to release from every cell in your body all unwanted memories, anxieties, pain and frustrations that are associated with this issue you have chosen to release. (Pause.)

Take a long, deep breath of release and hold the release statement (paper) in the flame of the candle and light it. Once the paper is lit, place it in the burning bowl to continue burning until it is done.

Be aware of what you are releasing. Be with it. Let it go. You no longer need that block in your life. You have learned from its experience and it is now time to move on in your life.

Next, light the sage and cedar and smudge yourself in whatever manner you choose.

Take the amethyst cluster in your left hand (your receiving hand). Allow the healing energies of the color vibration of purple / violet to begin filling up inside of you. Visualize the color violet surrounding you and breathe this into your lungs. Breathe violet into your inner being.

Allow the healing energies of the amethyst crystals to travel up
your left arm. Visualize the healing energies traveling down to
your heart center, your love center. The heart grows and expands
in love and healing light. It renews you. It revitalizes you.
See the healing energies traveling up to your right shoulder and
down your right arm. Direct the energy down to your right hand
and outward. This is your giving hand, the hand that sends and
directs energy outward. Be in tune with the healing energy going
into your left hand and out of your right hand. (Pause for three
minutes.)

Take the amethyst cluster and now place it in your right hand.
Again, be in tune with the energies of the crystal and your
visualization of the color violet. (Pause for three minutes.)

Place the crystal cluster against your chest at the heart center.
The points of the crystal are directed toward your body and both
hands are holding the crystal over your heart. You are now
completing the circuit of the energy flow. Attune to this
sensation. (Pause for three to five minutes.)

When you feel completed, place the amethyst in front of you.

Pick up the paper strips, pen and pad and write a simple, positive
statement. This can be something that you desire or are aiming
for in your life. Write it as an affirmation. When you have done
this, write the same statement on each of the other two remaining
papers.

Read each paper and fold it four times. Do this individually with
each paper. Take time to absorb what you have written.

Take each affirmation and place one on your left side, one on your
right side and one in front of you.

Take the one in front and place it on your meditation table, so
you will have it for future meditations.

Now, take the remaining two papers that are at your sides. Place one in your left (receiving) hand and the other in your right (giving) hand. Put both hands over your heart center.

Say the affirmation (that you have written) out loud. * Acknowledge what it is that you are welcoming into your life.

    also say:

" I receive and give to myself and others. I accept and share this manifestation in my life. "

Accept this to happen to you on all levels of your being: spiritual, causal, mental, astral, etheric and physical levels. (Pause.)

On completion of your meditation, take the two remaining papers and place one under your pillow and one in your pocket.

Do not mix up the papers. The energies will be different. One is coming to you on an unconscious level in your dream state. The other will come to you on a conscious level as you carry it with you and take it out to look at it daily.

This is a very, powerful meditation. May you prosper.

* If you are experiencing this exercise in a group setting, then you can just say your affirmation mentally.

Group   Alterations

- Everyone has a small amethyst cluster
- Use one central candle
- Use one central burning bowl
- One person smudges everyone and then the last person will smudge the " Smudger ".

(This meditation was channeled through me for my friend, Rev. Bella Salerno. She enjoyed participating in the ceremony.)

MY PERSONAL EXPERIENCE:

How To Do A House Blessing

There are many ways to do a house blessing. There are no set
rules. Be open to using your imagination and your creativity.
I went to visit the home of my massage therapist, Joya Verde. She
had her home designed and built in a nice country setting. This
was my first visit to Joya's new home. There is a tradition that
is shared by many cultures. When one visits another's new home,
during the initial visit, they bring a house warming gift. My
gift to Joya was a house blessing ceremony. What a great gift!
She joined me and together we shared in blessing her new home.

Optional supplies:

Prayer blanket, smudging supplies, holy water, five clear quartz
crystals (finger size or larger), tobacco or cornmeal, a purple,
votive candle and matches.

Joya and I began together outside in the direction of the
East. We set up the prayer blanket and made it a ground altar.
All of the supplies were placed on the altar for smudging and
blessing.

We began with an opening prayer.

" Father, Mother, Son as One: We bless this home and Joya.
We bless them that they will be a light unto others. We bless all
of those who come here that they may find their Inner Light. We
bless this sacred space that we create this day. We call on the
Four Directions. We call on those energies to support us in this
blessing. We ask that this blessing serve us and this sacred
space to our highest good. It is good. It is done. So be it."

The sage, cedar and sweetgrass were lit in an abalone shell.
I smudged and blessed all of the crystals to be used in the
ceremony. We began with the direction of the East and we smudged
the area. Next, we smudged the South, West and North of the
house. We returned to the East and began again. This time we
connected with the energies of the East and I planted a crystal
on the East side of the house. Joya sprinkled some blessed
tobacco on the spot. (Many Native Americans offer blessed
cornmeal or tobacco to the nature spirits of the area of where
they will live, work, seek a vision, dig a crystal, etc.)

161

We continued to connect with the remaining directions of the South, West and North. As I planted a crystal at each site, Joya, holding a purple candle accompanied me. (Purple is the color of transmutation. The violet flame of St. Germaine is transmutative. You can visualize working with this in your healing practice. During my session work, I place unwanted, discharged energies that have been released during the healing, into the violet flame. The violet vibration will transmute those energies into pure light.) We used the candle during the blessing to represent the Light of the Creator. Also note that in planting the crystals, I planted them with the point up. Some of the terminated end of the crystal was exposed.

After we did all of the four directions, I took the remaining crystal and used it to connect with each crystal site. I began with the East again and gently tapped the crystal point to the crystal planted in the earth. I visualized linking up each crystal with an etheric cord of energy, as I went to each crystal site. All of the four sites were linked up to each other. That action placed the house in the center of a vortex of energy.

After we had done all of the four directions of the house, we went to the entrance of the house. I placed a crystal under the steps. A prayer was said into the crystal. We placed into the crystal the intention that all who walk over it may find their Inner Light and be healed. Many people come to Joya for a healing in her service work.

The last phase of the ceremony, which is optional, is to use holy water and bless the four sites outside. The cleansing, water element is also used by sprinkling a little into each room, inside the house. A flick of the wrist will dispense a small amount into the center of each area.

We did a blessing on the inside of the house. Earlier when the smudging herbs were lit, we had also gone into the house and smudged each room. As I went around blessing the home with holy water, Joya went into each room with the candle. An affirmation was spoken to confirm that each room was cleared of any unwanted energies and was blessed.

A prayer was said for those who live in the home. The purple, votive candle was given to Joya. It was placed in her healing room. There is a sweat lodge on Joya's and Virginia's property. It was built by Morning Star. She had used sage and cedar for consecrating the ground. Many will continue to come to this sacred space to grow. The crystals will support this.

A Prayer of Release

" Divine Creator: Father, Mother Son as One: We ask for a Blessing of Release. We are open to a release between _____ and _____. Sever, cut, unbind, and release all unwanted thoughts, feelings and emotions. And it is done.... (slap hand together to represent cutting the etheric cord connection.) So be it. "

Candle of Release

I release into the Light any pain, any hurt that I may be feeling.

I release into the Light any anger, frustration, resentment or jealousy that I may be expressing.

I release any and all unwanted thoughts and feelings into the flame of Eternal Light. All of these energies are being transmuted now into pure light.

It is good. It is done. So be it.

Sphere   of   Transformation

One amethyst sphere is needed for this exercise.

Relax and center yourself.

Hold the amethyst sphere in both hands. Place the sphere at your root chakra (front or back position).   Go inside yourself. Sense this chakra center and how it feels to you.   What impressions do you get? Do you feel a sensation? Do you get a mental image that associates with what is going on in this area? The first chakra relates to survival issues. It also relates to how we deal with changes in our lives. It is the security center that makes one preoccupied with basic needs of food, clothing and shelter.   After you have tuned into the chakra center, you are ready for the next step.

Be aware of what you need to let go of to balance out this center. Breathe into the quartz sphere and release any unwanted thoughts and feelings that are associated with this area.   Continue your releasing breath until you feel complete at this center. Mentally clear the quartz sphere and go to the second chakra.

Tune in to this center. This center relates to emotional issues. This center is about how we relate to the world in a sexual way. It is the sensation center and the center of creativity and reproduction. Do you relate with others from this space, or more from your heart center? What do you need to clear from this area? Do the Releasing Breath to balance out this center. When you are done, mentally clear the quartz sphere and go to the <u>remaining</u> chakras.

The third chakra, the solar plexus, is the power center.   It relates to how we represent ourselves to the world and our outward manifestations. It has to do with issues of will power. Is the energy coming from this center domineering, weak, or in balance?

The fourth chakra, the heart, is the center of compassion, the love center. Do you hold back sharing your love with others? Do you love yourself?

The fifth chakra, the throat, is the center of communication and expression. Are there words that you need to express to others? Do you share your truth?

The sixth chakra, the brow center, relates to clear seeing.

The seventh chakra, the crown, is a spiritual center that relates to pure knowing.

After you have done a reading on each chakra center and have cleared them, remove the sphere from your energy field. Place both of your palm chakras over the heart center. Feel the heart chakra coming into balance. (Pause for five minutes.)

Keep your left hand over your heart center. Place your right hand any place else that you feel guided. Send healing love to that area and feel it come into balance. See this area well, balanced and whole. Continue directing healing energy to other parts of your body, until you feel the session has come to an end.

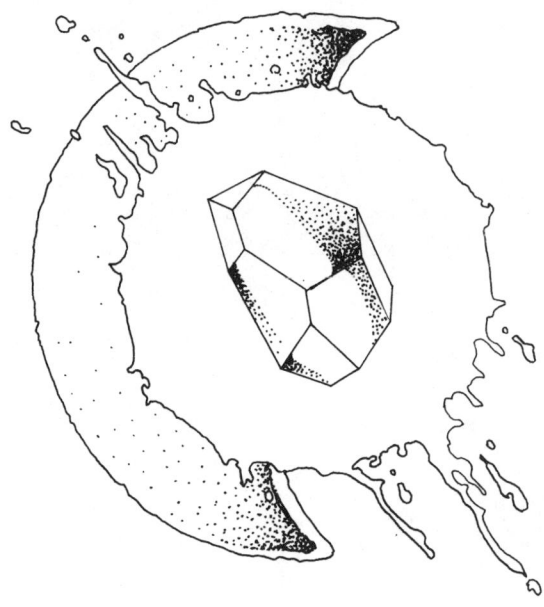

MY PERSONAL EXPERIENCE:

Partings   by   Ojela   Frank   10/30/81

Why is it so painful
to say good bye, sometimes?
Especially, to some one whom
you hold close in your heart?

You part and go
your own separate ways
and on occasion,
you find the opportunity
to come together again.

It is especially difficult,
if your relationship with each other
is kept at a distance.
Your moments together are rare.
So, you both treasure them,
instead of take them
for granted.

And when you depart,
you feel mixed emotions.
The joys, the highs
are experienced
from that person
making you feel special,
just by him or her loving you.

But also,
the sorrow is felt
and the fear
no longer can stay subsided.

The questions arise:
" Will we ever meet again? "
" Will we be able to share once more
what we just experienced? "
" Will God grant us this? "

Only time will tell.

So, you smile
and you cry
at the same time.

THE   HOLY   SACRAMENTS   and   CRYSTALS

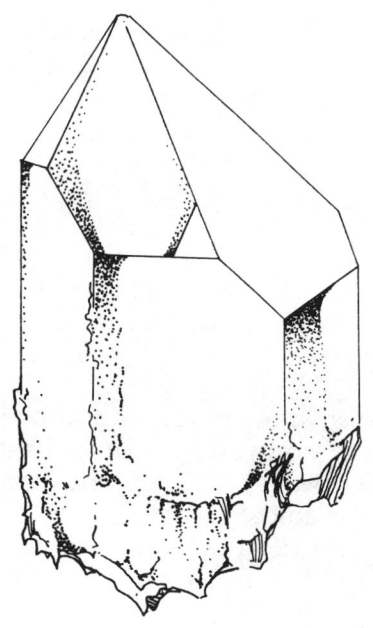

Last Fall, while visiting a friend in Virginia Beach, a favor was asked of me. Dorian, the editor of my books wanted to have a memorial service for her son who had recently passed away. She asked if I would facilitate a service that would support her. Her son had been cremated and she wanted to return his ashes to the earth, by way of the ocean. On the day of the event, a small group of friends came to support Dorian. I brought a few basic supplies and channeled the ceremony as it all took place. The whole experience was wonderful and very healing for all who shared in the event. I thank Dorian, Joy, Helen, Kathy and John for their openness and sharing. The following is a summary of what took place; you may want to share it with others some day.

RELEASING   CEREMONY
(Memorial   Service)

People who are to participate may gather. Bring a large number of small, clear quartz crystals. You'll need one per person to give out during the ceremony.

Create a sacred space.

   a. Set up a prayer blanket with crystals. Everyone will sit in a circle with the prayer blanket in the center.

   b. Light sage and cedar in an abalone shell for smudging. Pass the smudge shell counter clockwise for clearing the space. Each person will hold the shell in one hand and use the other hand to direct the incense smoke to different areas of his / her energy field. Also smudge the container of crystals.

   c. Sing or chant a song together to build up the vibration of the group.

The group will be in silence together for a short while. (If this releasing ceremony is including cremation ashes, place the container on the prayer blanket in the center of the group.

170

The immediate relatives may want to share a thought or a writing with the group. (There are two excellent readings found in Kahlil Gibran's, The Prophet. One reading is on death. Another reading is on children.) Everyone else in the group may take turns sharing a thought about the loved one and life.

More silence... (when it feels appropriate, the group will hold hands together and walk down to the ocean (or other site for releasing the ashes or burying the ashes.) Then the group returns in silence to sit in a circle once again around the prayer blanket.

Pass around the container of small crystals. Each person will choose one. Pause for silence. Each person will hold the crystal and put into it what he or she wants to release at this time: thoughts, feelings, etc. Each person directs what he or she wants to release into the crystal. When the link has been made, each person will go down to the ocean water individually and throw his or her crystal into the ocean or bury it in the earth. Return to the circle and meditate on what you just let go.

Facilitator: once everyone has released his or her crystal, you may choose to smudge the group or use Tibetan Tingsha bells to clear the energy fields of each person. This can be done quickly by going counter clockwise around the group with smudge smoke or the bells.

Facilitator: you may go around to anoint each person with a special attunement oil or holy water. Inner guidance will direct you as to exact placement of oil: on the brow center, heart center, or elsewhere. You may choose to visualize surrounding others with violet light or the violet flame of Saint Germaine for transmuting energies that have been released.

171

Sit in silence. If there are more crystals left over in the container, each person can be given one. This time each person will direct healing energy into the crystal. Each person may choose to put an affirming thought into the crystal. Then everyone will hold the crystal in both hands over the heart area. Each can visualize this affirmation or goal coming true in his or her life. Each may pray that this request may serve him or her to the highest good. Everyone will put the crystal in his or her pocket.

Facilitator: you may take a crystal and touch each person at the heart center linking the energies of each person in the group together, as one. When you have connected with everyone, including yourself, return the crystal to Mother Earth by throwing it into the ocean, or burying it in the ground.

Then the group may stand and join hands together and end the circle with a song and hugging each other.

One suggestion: " We are one in the infinite sun forever and ever and ever. "

Blessings.

A   NEW   AGE   CHRISTENING

CEREMONY for a NEW AGE CHRISTENING

As more and more babies are being born in the home, it is now appropriate to also do baptisms in the home.

Supplies: quartz crystals, anointing oils, holy water from a sacred place, smudging herbs: sage, cedar and sweetgrass, cassette player, sea salt, prayer blanket or altar table, four candles, matches, Angel Cards and sacred ashes. The ashes can be from a purification ceremony, Sai Baba's " vibhuti dust ", or from a Sacred Fire. Any of these supplies are optional. You may be guided to bring other items.

Preparations: Make an energy connection with the child you are going to christen. This can be done in person or with a photograph. Listen to what the parents have to share with you about the child. As you get an idea of the personality of the child, you will be able to attune finely to what crystal you will give as a spiritual gift.

Once you have selected a crystal for the child, cleanse it and program it. You can say a prayer into the crystal: " Let this crystal serve _____ to his / her highest good. "

If you have a photo, you can place the crystal on it to continue your energy connection until the day of the christening. Each time you go near the photo, you can say a short prayer asking for guidance. Each child is unique and has personal spiritual needs. If you have made some sort of energy connection with the child ahead of time, you'll be guided as to what supplies you'll need for the ceremony. You'll also be guided to what actions you'll need to do during the ceremony for the child's personal growth.

It is important to make a connection ahead of time with one or both of the parents. If you have a counseling or healing practice, a session will bond you closer together. This will make the whole experience more intimate and rewarding for all involved.

If there is a small gathering of people for the christening, you can offer to do a blessing of the group towards the end of the ceremony. A nice gift would be to share with everyone there a small crystal point or tumbled stone of quartz. The friends and relatives will feel a closer bonding taking place in being an active part of the ceremony. You can ask ahead of time, the number of guests expected for the event. Small points or tumbled stones are inexpensive and are much appreciated by all. Smudge the environment with burning herbs of sage and cedar.

Set up a prayer blanket or a table as an altar. You may choose to place on the altar / blanket various crystals, an altar candle, gemstones and sacred objects. Large generator size crystals or clusters can be placed at the four directions of the blanket or in the center of the room. Here are some suggestions:

Four large, clear quartz crystals with the points directed into the center, each point located at the four directions. Start with placing the first crystal in the direction of the East. Then place the other crystals in the directions of the South, West and North. If the crystals are generators, the points can be aimed up.

Four large clusters as described above. You can mix different types of quartz: clear quartz, amethyst, citrine quartz, smoky quartz, a large " Herkimer Diamond " quartz, a large chunk of rose quartz, blue or green quartz. These are some of the suggestions. You will feel guided as to what is appropriate for the child's energy.

Some suggested patterns for crystal layouts are:

The Four Directions.

A Star of David (as described in Frank Alper's Exploring Atlantis Vol. I).

A circle pattern. You can attune to how many crystals and what combination will be appropriate for the ceremony. One nice combination is alternating a clear quartz, rose quartz, clear quartz, rose quartz pattern.

The following is a list of the stages of the Rites of a Baptism / Christening:

The reception of the Child

A sharing of a sacred reading

Spiritual Cleansing

Anointing before Baptism

Celebration of the Sacrament

Blessing

Invocation

Baptism

Anointing after Baptism

Lighted Candle Connection

Conclusion of the Rite

Blessing of the group and dismissal

Upon arrival in the home:

Smudge the environment.

Get out all of the supplies and set up a sacred space.

As the guests arrive, you can have mellow music playing on a tape recorder to quiet everyone down. It helps to set the mood.

THE   CEREMONY

Begin with a Group Circle holding hands. Say a prayer of thanks for the sharing that is taking place. Give a few minutes for quiet reflection and meditation.

Reception of the Child:

Godparents or parents come forward with the child. As they hold the child, make a Sign of the Cross on the forehead. If you feel guided to, you can say a prayer.

Sharing of sacred readings:

A nice reading from the Bible is John 3: verses 3 through 8:

3   " Jesus answered: " I am telling you the truth: no one can see the Kingdom of God unless he is born again. "

4   " How can a grown man be born again? " Nicodemus asked.
" He certainly cannot enter his mother's womb and be born a second time! "

5   " I am telling you the truth, " replied Jesus, " that no one can enter the Kingdom of God unless he is born of water and the Spirit. 6 A person is born physically of human parents, but he is born spiritually of the Spirit. 7 Do not be surprised because I tell you that you must all be born again. 8 The wind blows wherever it wishes; you hear the sound it makes, but you do not know where it comes from or where it is going. It is like that with everyone who is born of the Spirit. "

(Other readings from the Bible are listed at the end of the chapter.)   Another reading could be from the teachings of Lao Tzu.   Here is one from <u>The Way of Life According to Lao Tzu</u>:

Reading # 6:

The breath of life moves through a deathless valley
Of mysterious motherhood
Which conceives and bears the universal seed,
The seeming of a world never to end,
Breath for men to draw from as they will:
And the more they take of it, the more remains.

                                                                                    2.

Another suggested reading: A Reading on Children by Kahlil Gibran's <u>The Prophet</u>.

Something that I shared:

" Birth is an initiation.   As we go throughout life, we experience many initiations, many awakenings. "

Exorcism / Spiritual Cleansing:

Smudge the child with sage and cedar.

Anointing before Baptism:

Anoint the child on the breast with cedar oil.

Celebration of the Sacrament:

Blessing and Invocation:

" In Baptism we use water to symbolize the gift of grace in this sacrament. This water reminds us of when Jesus was baptized in the river Jordan by John the Baptist. By the power of the Holy Spirit give the water the sharing of your Divine Essence. Cleanse this child in Love, Light, Truth and Wisdom by the water and the Spirit. (Celebrant touches the water with the right hand.)

" Divine Creator, we ask for a blessing to sanctify this child, body and soul through water. We ask that you fill this child's new life with abundance, joy peace and love. We ask that you give him / her grace as he / she learns to walk his / her own spiritual path. We ask that you guide this child well with your Light. "

Baptism:

Take the Holy Water and make the symbol of a triangle on the forehead. (The triangle is an ancient symbol that represents Light.)

Take salt and make the symbol of a square on the chin.
(This earthly sign represents the support of strength and firmness that is needed on the earth plane.)

Take ash and make the Sign of the Cross on the breast.
(This signifies the power of sacrifice and love that should grow in the human heart.)

3.

Make the Sign of the Cross over the child three times.

" I baptize you in the name of the Trinity. (Father, Son and Holy Spirit or Father, Mother, Son as One.)

Anointing after Baptism:

Anoint the crown (top of the head) with oil. (You may also feel guided to anoint other chakra points.)

Lighted Candle Connection:

Both parents have a candle each and will light a third candle together. They light their child's candle.

" Receive the Light of God. You are keepers of the Light.
Let this be a remembrance that you always carry the Divine Spark.
It is your Divine purpose to share your Light by example of
thoughts, words and actions. You are the first teachers of your
child. It is by your examples that your child will grow and be
formed. "

Blessing of the child's eyes, ears and mouth.

Blessing of the child's crystal. (Give the crystal in a pouch
to the parents to place in the baby's crib.)

Blessing of the mother and child.

Blessing of the father and child.

Blessing of the family. (Give a quartz cluster to the family as
a spiritual gift.)

" By God's gift through water and the Holy Spirit we are
reborn to everlasting life. "

Blessing of the group. (Give a small crystal to each guest.)

Group sharing: This is a good time for guests to share a blessing
or an affirmation for the parents and child. Ask the guests if
they have anything to share.

Closing prayer.

Dismissal.

Here is a summary of events for the ceremony that can fit onto an index card:

Altar set up: light candle

Open Circle

Reception of Child

    Sign of the Cross on the FOREHEAD

Readings: Bible (John 3 verse 3 - 8)

Spiritual Cleansing: anointing before Baptism
    smudge with sage and cedar, cedar oil on BREAST

Celebration

    Blessing and Invocation

    Baptism:

    WATER on the FOREHEAD = TRIANGLE   = Light

    SALT on the CHIN   = SQUARE   = strength & earth

    ASH   on the BREAST   = CROSS   = sacrifice & love

Sign of the Cross three times over child

Anointing after Baptism: oil on CROWN

LIGHTED CANDLES: (1) altar candle (lighted at the beginning)
(2) parents (1) child

Blessing of the child's eyes, ears and mouth

Gift of crystal to child

Blessing of mother & child, father & child, family

Gift of crystal cluster to the family

Gift of crystals to the group

Blessing of group & sharing

Closing prayer.

Here are some recommended readings from the Bible for those who want a more Christian oriented ceremony:

John 3: verses 3 - 8

Acts 2: verses 36 - 39

Titus 3: verses 4 -7

John 14: verse 23

1st Corinthians 3: verse 6, also verse 16

1st Peter 2: verse 9

Matthew 28: verses 18 - 20

Notes:

1. American Bible Society, Good News Bible: Today's English Version, (New York: ABS, 1977), p. 126 - 127.

2. Witter Bynner, The Way of Life According to Lao Tzu, (New York: Capricorn Books, 1962), p. 28.

3. Stanley Drake, The Path to Birth, (Edinburgh, Great Britain: Floris Books, 1979), p. 62.

Other recommended books for researching your own style of ceremony are:

Christian Minister's Manual, which can be obtained from the National Chaplain's Association in Florida. They have a toll free number.

Rites of Baptism by the National Conference of Bishops of the U.S., Liturgical Press, Collegeville, Minn.

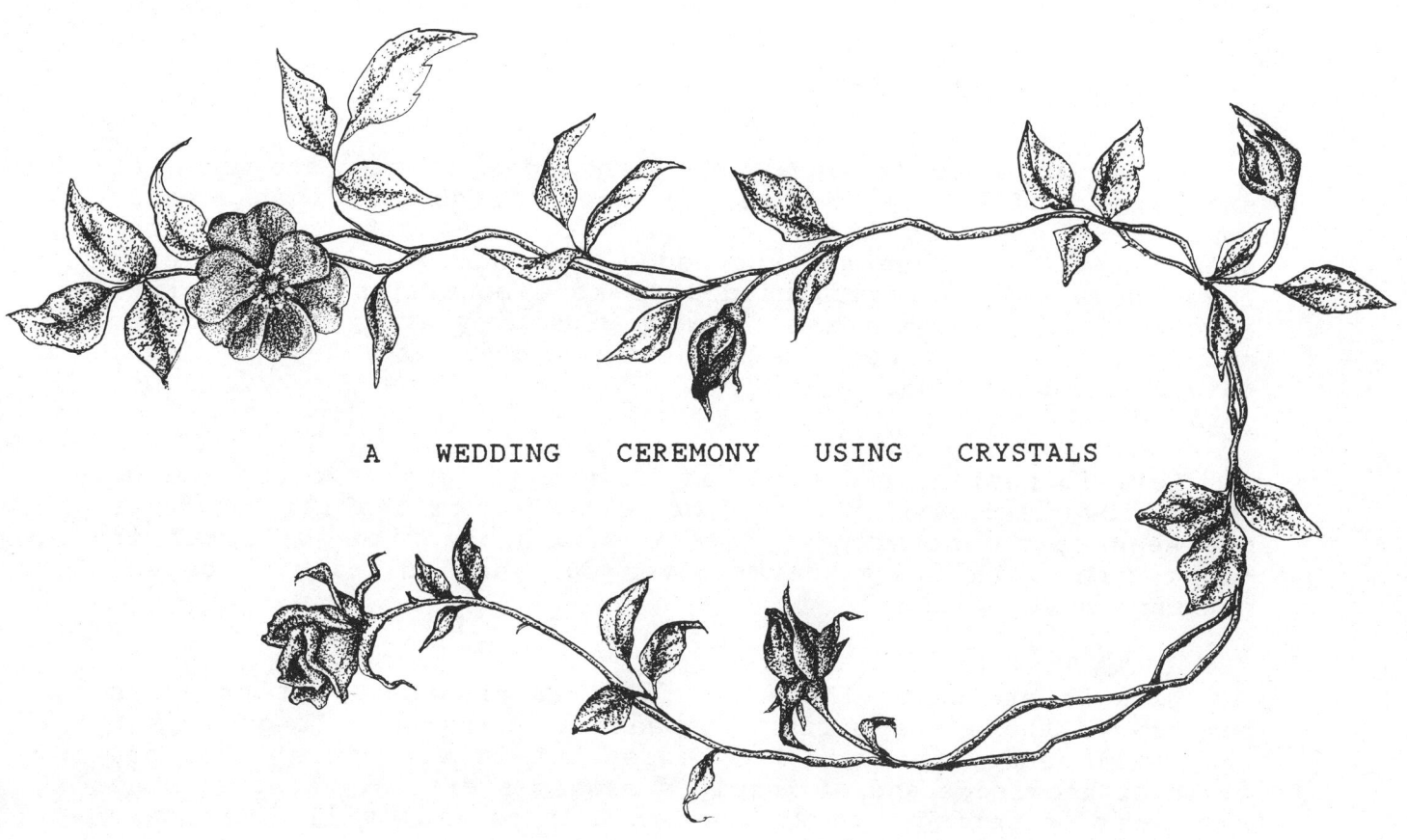

A   WEDDING   CEREMONY   USING   CRYSTALS

Reading   from   the   New   Testament

from 1 Corinthians: Verse 13

    I may be able to speak the languages of men and even of
angels, but if I have no love, my speech is no more than a noisy
gong or a clanging bell. I may have the gift of inspired
preaching; I may have all knowledge and understand all secrets;
I may have all the faith needed to move mountains... but, if I
have no love, I am nothing. I may give away everything I have,
and even give up my body to be burned... but, if I have no love,
this does me no good.

    Love is patient and kind; it is not jealous or conceited or
proud; love is not ill-mannered or selfish or irritable; love does
not keep record of wrongs; love is not happy with evil, but is
happy with Truth. Love never gives up; and its faith, hope and
patience never fail.

    Love is eternal. There are inspired messages, but they are
temporary; there are gifts of speaking in strange tongues, but
they will cease; there is knowledge, but it will pass. For our
gifts of knowledge and of inspired messages are only partial; but
when what is perfect comes, then what is partial will disappear.

    When I was a child, my speech, feelings and thinking were all
those of a child; now that I am a man, I have no more use for
childish ways. What we see now is like a dim image in a mirror;
then we shall see face-to-face. What I know now is only partial;
then it will be complete... as complete as God's knowledge of me.

    Meanwhile, these three remain: faith, hope and love; and the
greatest of these is love.

                                              1.

SELECTED   READINGS   ON   LOVE,   FRIENDSHIP   &   MARRIAGE

A friend is one to whom
one may pour out all the
contents of one's heart,
chaff and grain together,
knowing that the gentlest
of hands will take and
sift it, keep what is worth
keeping and, with the
breath of kindness, blow
the rest away.

Arabian   proverb

The spaces are everywhere.
My space is here.
Your space is there.
But, the bonding motion of love
joins two together
as if contained
in only one space.

Ojela

Love that does not renew
itself every day
becomes a habit
and in turn, a slavery.

Kahlil Gibran   2.

Beyond the illusions
going deeply inward,
I see inside of you
touching you
knowing you
and loving what I see and feel.
Your response
is so in tune with mine.
We are touching souls
as soulmates.
The Universe
is our playground
and it echoes
of our rejoicing.

                    Ojela Frank

May the sky rain peace
and the Earth grow love.
We shall dance
in between
forever.

                         Diana

Today I reached out
to you
across the miles...
the love I held
for you
brought you
here by my side
to comfort me.

                    Ojela

WEDDING   VOWS: by Ojela Frank

Life is always constantly changing.   I will continue to
change, as will you.   As I go throughout life, I will share with
you my changes, growths and learnings.

I will give to you my best effort all of the time, in being
your friend, lover, companion, wife, mother of our children, a
sister and a mother to you, when you need a mother image to
comfort you.   I give to you my best, and if the moments come that
I do not live up to this, then I ask that you gently remind me.

We have touched souls.   We have felt and shared our essences
within each other, and will continue to do so in life, as it
unfolds for us and we journey down its path.

I see the beauty within you, the God within you and I share
with you also, mine in return.   We are only a fraction of God's
Plan, God's Being.   Together we will know and share this with
others.   For the World is our family, the Universe, our
playground.   And we will take each day together and grow in that
image.

WEDDING   VOWS: by Eugene   Frank

I promise to hold you in love. This loving will be not only
in words but, by my actions toward you and for you. I will love
you through whatever life will bring. I will be with you holding
you in love in the sunshine or darkness, whatever life will bring.

My hope is that our love will grow each day, for love can
never stand still. Love must go forward, or retreat. And I hope
that hand in hand, we can go forward in life and love together.

May this Circle of Love that we solemnize this day, lead us
to love each other increasingly, and be the means for loving all
God has chosen for us to love. I hold you in love and the Light
of Christ.

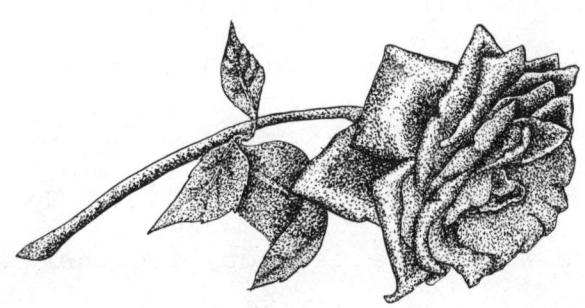

I know that if I offer
my friendship to all
as Christ did,
I shall begin to feel
the Cosmic love
which is God.

Paramahansa Yogananda   3.

We are an oasis
to one another
having traveled
in emotional droughts;
we now sip
from each other's love cup
filled to the brim
and overflowing.

Ojela Frank

How Do I Love Thee?

How do I love thee? Let me count the ways.
I love thee to the depth and breadth and height
My soul can reach, when feeling out of sight
For the ends of Being an ideal Grace.
I love thee to the level of everyday's
Most quiet need, by sun and candle-light.
I love thee freely, as men strive for Right;
I love thee purely, as they turn from Praise.
I love thee with the passions put to use
In my old griefs, and with my childhood's faith.
I love thee with a love I seemed to lose
With my lost saints, I love thee with the breath,
Smiles, tears, of all my life! And, if God choose,
I shall but love thee better after death.

Elizabeth Barrett Browning
4.

We are spiritual lovers.
We are emotional lovers.
Physically, we are also friends.
You kiss my hand.
I kiss your face all over.
Our love interplays
the energy is felt
coming from
and being sent
to each other.

As my love for you
grows
expands
transcends
I feel you.

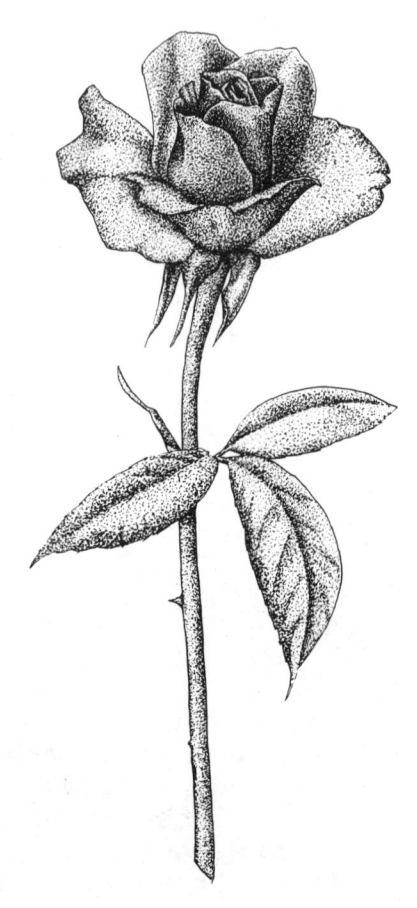

In the evenings,
I feel you close by
As I hug my pillow,
or my teddy bear.
I embrace you fondly
wanting
and needing
your responses of love
in return.

I love you.
I miss you.
I need you.
And some day,
I pray that
we may take
each day,
moment by moment
and share
life's joys and treasures
together.

                    Ojela   Frank

<u>Love Is</u>   by Ojela Frank   2/9/72

Love is tender
and kind.
It's like an eternal flame
always burning deeply in your heart.

Love is truth
and real.
It's so strong
that it overpowers your mind, body and soul.

Love... is for giving
and keeping.
It's something to treasure
and always cherish.

Love is inspiration
and passion.
It's a feeling
of want and need.
Love is to share
and care.

Love is an outstretched hand
to all
of your brothers and sisters.

Love is faith
and hope.
Someday
it will spread to all.

Navajo   Prayer

When you were children, you talked like children,
But now that you've grown, you should be done
with childish things and put them away.
When you were children, you looked into a mirror
that gave only a blurred reflection of reality.
But with love and maturity, you shouldn't be
afraid to look into that mirror and see each
other face to face.
Be swift like the wind in loving each other.
Be brave like the sea in loving each other.
Be gentle like the breeze in loving each other.
Be patient like the sun who waits and watches
the four changes of the Earth in loving each other.
Be wise like the roaring of the thunder clouds
and lightning in loving each other.
Be shining like the morning dawn in loving each other.
Be proud like the tree who stands without bending
in loving each other.
Be brilliant like the rainbow colors in loving each other.
Now, forever, forever, there will be no more loneliness,
because your worlds are joined together with the world.
Forever, forever.

                                                5.

A Song by Ojela Frank

For the Rest of My Life   9/1/80

All my life I've searched
For the right thing to do.
Another day goes by
And I share it all with You.
For You came into my life
At a time when I needed You the most.
A Friend like you, I can hold onto
For the rest of my life.

Times are hard, but with You
My troubles are so few.
You take care of my daily life
Since I gave it all up to You.
Days go on
Yes, they come and go.
And I see that You never really change.
A Friend like You, I can hold onto
For the rest of my life.

You brought sunshine to me
At the darkest depths I've ever known.
You picked me up, off the ground
And You lifted up my soul.
All because I opened my door
And I let You come within.
A Friend like You, I can hold onto
For the rest of my life.

Wedding   Preparations

It is important to meet with the couple prior to the wedding.
This will give you an opportunity to get to know the couple. It
will also give you an idea of their needs.

Does the couple want a traditional wedding? If so, of what
faith? As an Interfaith Minister, I am able to partake in doing
ceremonies with other clergy members of a traditional practice.
Many interfaith weddings have two ministers to support the bride
and groom. I am also authorized to do weddings by myself outside
of the traditional style.

Does the couple want the wedding indoors or outdoors? If the
wedding is not to be a traditional ceremony, what kind of things
would the couple like to take place?

I am writing about doing my first wedding. The opportunity
came to me, while I was writing this book. Elisabeth Lindberg,
a massage therapist and her fiance, Tom Baldwin, a pilot
approached me. Both had been married before and have children
from previous marriages. Both Elisabeth and Tom were open to my
doing a New Age style of wedding ceremony for them.

When the couple came for counseling, they were unclear about
the particulars that they wanted included in the ceremony. They
were busy being in love with each other. There were stars in
their eyes. The love they shared for each other was powerful.
By the end of our sharing, it was clear that I was going to be in
charge of creating a ceremony for the both of them. This was a
challenge for me. I did much contemplation and meditation to see
what I would be guided to come up with. I share this with you
now.

Supplies:

Selected Readings on the subject of love and marriage

- 1 Corinthians: Verse 13

- The Prophet by Kahlil Gibran: on Love, on Marriage,
  on Friendship

- Shakespeare: Sonnets 56, 115

- readings from a Course in Miracles (the text)

196

Supplies continued:

- Sound instruments: Tibetan bells and bowls, tape recorder and music tapes for selected music.

- Attunement oils, Holy Water, and other tools for blessing the couple.

- Prayer Blanket for the altar or ground

- Quartz crystal and minerals for ceremony or grid work, also for giving out to the guests.

- Wedding rings

- Ceremony outline

- Wedding candles: two thin taper candles and one large one for the Lighting Ceremony.

- Wedding document: to be signed by witnesses. You'll find a sample of one in this chapter.

- Marriage License: must be signed by the minister and two witnesses. It is the responsibility of the minister to see that the license and the blood test results are sent to the state / county authorities in the area that the wedding takes place.

- Honeymoon candle: a white, six day votive candle. The couple takes the candle with them on their honeymoon. Once the couple arrives at their destination, the candle remains lit for the week.

Wedding   Ceremony   Outline

The bride and groom wear crystal pouches for one month prior to
the wedding. On the wedding day, they will exchange crystal
pouches. Each one contains the energy of the other. They will
carry the essence of each other's presence when they are apart.

Pre-cleanse: Bride and Groom take an individual, spiritual
cleansing bath with water, sea salt and apple cider vinegar. This
is a preparation for the ceremony and spiritual initiation.

Music: Tape recorder (battery operated) and selected tape
recordings of mellow music to help set the mood. Popular
suggestion: Pachelbel's Canon and also the Fairy Ring.

Set up a Crystal Pattern and Meditation Altar: If outdoors, you
can create a ground altar using a prayer blanket. Make the
crystal pattern large enough for the couple to stand inside later.
Connect with the energies of each of the Four Directions. Begin
with the East, then the South, West, North and return to the East
position. You may choose to smudge your altar space along with
the Four Direction connection. Next, take a crystal or cluster
and make an energy connection with the East direction. Take
another crystal and connect with the South direction and so on.
You are creating an energy field that the couple will stand
together in during the ceremony. Place on the altar space the
other supplies that will be used during the ceremony.

Smudging Supplies: After the bride and groom have come together
at the beginning of the ceremony, you can smudge them both with
sage, cedar and sweetgrass.

Read the actual ceremony that is included in this chapter. It
explains things well. For additional notes, see below:

Attunement: You can use special healing oils. Anoint both the
bride and groom with the oil on their foreheads. You can rub the
oil in your hands and stroke their energy fields in a downward or
a swirling motion. You are helping to balance their energies.
Do both the front and back of the energy fields. This attunement
process is done prior to the bride and groom entering the crystal
grid pattern. When they are in the energy grid work, they will
be even more open with each other from this balancing process.
You also could apply the oils to an Atlantean Healing Paddle and
use as described above. (See Frank Alper's Exploring Atlantis
Vol. III for more description on the energy paddles.)

Playing of the Tibetan Bells and Temple Bowls: You can play these sound healing instruments for all to enjoy. Walk around the couple a few times as you play different types of bells. I also played a silver tinker bell. I shook the little bell over the crown chakras of the bride and groom. It was also played in a circular motion around their heads and necks.

Children's Blessing: This was not the initial wedding for Tom and Elisabeth. Both of them together have seven children. We wanted to do something in the ceremony that would include the children. As I look back and remember the day of their wedding, one of the most memorable events was the connection of the parents with the circle of children. This segment of the ceremony took place after the couple was married, but played an active part in the ceremony. Both Tom and Elisabeth remained in the center of their crystal grid pattern, while the children surrounded them in a circle. Both parents looked silently together at each child, one by one. They kept their eyes connected until the energy exchange felt complete. A lot of love was exchanged back and forth in the parent - children circle. Once the parents had connected with each child, I introduced them as one new family to the wedding guests.

Lastly, a crystal was given to each wedding guest and we all shared in a blessing of the couple and the group together.

Because the wedding ceremony took place outside, we saved the Lighting of the Wedding Candle until the wedding reception. A reading was shared on the Lighting of the Wedding Candle. To support this action, I gave the couple a Honeymoon Candle. It was a white, six day votive candle. They took it on their honeymoon to Tahiti. The candle remained lit for the remainder of the week. As they looked at it, they were reminded of their special day together. They took my reading on the lighting ceremony with them.

It was also nice to watch different guests signing the Wedding Document that Erica made. The document will some day be framed and displayed on the Baldwin's wall. I also gave the couple a marriage certificate that I purchased in a religious supply store. They said they were going to frame it along with the State Marriage License.

All in all, this was a very special experience. I am thankful to be a part of it. I invite any other ministers of New Age philosophy to use this ceremony in their wedding services, if they feel guided to do so. My next wedding ceremony will be a lot easier to do, now that I have this outline to follow.

Summary of a Wedding Ceremony

1) Entrance / Procession

   Greeting to the Bride, Groom and witnesses

   Opening Prayer

2) Liturgy of the Word

3) Homily / Sermon

4) Rite of Marriage

   Consent / Vows

   Exchange of Rings

5) Nuptial Blessing

6) Pronouncement

7) Conclusion / Blessing

A NEW AGE WEDDING CEREMONY

Music playing: Pachelbel's Canon

Entrance: Bride was escorted down the path by her two eldest sons.

Declaration of Consent:

To Groom: Thomas Baldwin, will you have this woman to be your wife? If so, answer, " I will. "

To Bride: Elisabeth Lindberg, will you have this man to be your husband? If so, answer, " I will. "

Giving of the Bride:

To escorts: Who is giving this woman to be married to this man? (Escorts answer " We do. ")

Bride is presented to the groom.

Greeting:

" Tom and Elisabeth, you have come together this day so that God may seal and strengthen your love in the presence of all your loved ones here. We support you both in love and in friendship."

Smudge the bride and groom, wedding rings, crystal grid, altar or prayer blanket and objects to be used for the ceremony. This is a form of spiritual cleansing done with sage, cedar and sweetgrass.

Opening Prayer:

" Divine Creator: Father, Mother, Son as One, hear our prayers for Elisabeth and Tom, who today are united in marriage before your altar of nature. Give them your blessing and strengthen their love for each other. "

Reading from the New Testament: (optional)

1 Corinthians: Verse 13   " Love is... "

Gospel reading from the Bible: (optional)

2 John: Verse 1 - 11 The Marriage Feast of Cana

A shared saying:

" Everyone who loves is born of God and knows him. "
            (1 John: Verse 4 - 7)

Related Readings:

                A friend is one to whom
                one may pour out all the
                contents of one's heart,
                chaff and grain together,
                knowing with the gentlest
                of hands will take and
                sift it, keep what is worth
                keeping and, with the
                breath of kindness, blow
                the rest away.

                    An Arabian proverb

A Reading on Friendship: by Kahlil Gibran from <u>The Prophet</u>.

Attunement Oils and Energy Balancing & Blessing

Couple enters the crystal grid work.

A Reading on Love: by Kahlil Gibran from <u>The Prophet</u>.

Consent / Vows: (Repeated after the minister:)

    " I, Thomas Arthur Baldwin, take you, Berit Elisabeth Lindberg
to be my wife and guiding companion, to have and to hold, from
this day forward. I promise to love you, comfort you, honor and
keep you in sickness and in health, in hard times as well as the
good times. I welcome God into our holy covenant of marriage now
and forever. "

" I, Berit Elisabeth Lindberg, take you, Thomas Arthur Baldwin, to be my husband and guiding companion, to have and to hold from this day forward. I promise to love you, comfort you, honor and keep you in sickness and in health, in hard times as well as the good times. I welcome God into our holy covenant of marriage now and forever. "

Minister: " And now, Thomas and Elisabeth would like to share with you their personal wedding vows to each other. "

Reading on Wedding Rings by Rev. Ojela Frank

Blessing of the Rings: (You may use holy water.)

   " May the Divine Creator bless these rings, which you give to each other as the sign of your love and fidelity. "

The bride and groom separately repeat the following saying after the minister, while placing the ring on the other's finger:

   " I give you this ring, as a symbol of my vow, and with all that I am and all that I have, I honor you. "

6.

Pronouncement of Marriage:

   " Therefore, by virtue of the authority vested in me as a minister of God and in accordance with the laws of God and the sovereign state of New Jersey, I now pronounce you husband and wife. What God has joined together, let man not separate. "

Nuptial Kiss:

Minister: " You may kiss the bride. "

Reading on Marriage by Kahlil Gibran from The Prophet.

Nuptial Blessing:

" Divine Creator: Father, Mother, Son as One, we ask that you bless Tom and Elisabeth this day and always. Assist them in their relationship with each other. Be their guiding Light to help them find and know their inner Light and Truth. Be with them always, so that they may know and feel your presence. Journey with them together, so that they may feel the oneness of whom they can become. Support them so you can be their Foundation and Strength. As their love grows together, strengthen it, so that it expands and they know no limitations. We ask this in your presence. Amen. "

Playing of Tibetan Temple Bells & Singing Bowls.

Reading on Children by Kahlil Gibran from <u>The Prophet</u>.

Children Blessing: (optional)

The children gather around their parents to form a circle. They join hands and support their parents by sending them loving thoughts. The parents together look at each child, one at a time. When they feel the energy exchange complete with each child, they then leave the crystal grid work. They join the circle with the children holding hands. They are united as one new family.

Presentation of the Newlyweds & Family

Group Blessing"

Each wedding guest receives a small quartz crystal.

" May these crystals be a reminder that you were present this day in love and friendship. Let them remind you that you support Tom and Elisabeth in their marriage and their love for each other. I bless you all in Light, Love and Truth. Go in peace. Amen. "

<u>A Reading On Wedding Rings</u> by Rev. Ojela Frank

Rings are a symbol of oneness. Two, living separate lives, come together as one. Each cares for the other so much, that they choose to share their lives together with one another. Each ring represents one's separate life. When they are placed together, they are intertwined in binding love and unite as one. Together they symbolize oneness. Each is separate and strong in one's own foundation and yet, at the same time, both are aspects of one vibration. Both are aspects of oneness. It is the attunement to love that creates the realization of oneness and unity. In the love vibration, there is expansion beyond self and there is unity with all.

Each ring represents a circle of love, and when combined, embraces and becomes one circle of love expanded even greater. It has been a choice of free will that these two have chosen to come together in a conscious decision, to share their lives together as one. Thus, they make their strong foundation even stronger. When two share as one, there is complete sharing, complete openness and no separation.

When two conscious souls come together to share as one, they are aware that it is important to be interdependent upon one another. That is perfect balance. If one is too dependent upon the other, it becomes a strain upon the relationship. Especially, for the one who is fulfilling the needs of the one who is dependent. On the other hand, if both are too independent, then there is not a touching stone. There is not a base for them to stay connected. The two independent beings continue to drift apart over a period of time. So, in the dance and interplay of being interdependent, one is free to dance a separate life and come back and dance together with the other.

The rings are blessed as one and yet they are worn separately. But when the two souls come together and embrace, they again unite with the symbol of a greater love. Two beings that become one. We are all one. We are all love.

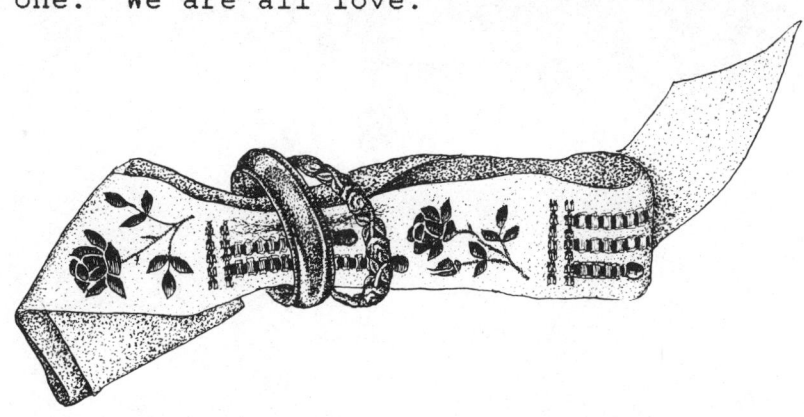

A Reading On the Lighting of the Wedding Candles

by Rev. Ojela Frank

The lighting of two separate candles represents two beings coming from two separate lives. As they unite together to light one candle, they become one in their energies. These people have chosen to combine their gifts, their lives together and become one energy vibration, one expanded unit of love.

There is no separation, only illusion that there is separation. We are love. We are light. When one is aware of these energies, they are aware of expanded consciousness beyond the boundary of their physical body. These two souls have chosen to walk the path of Oneness.

Today's ceremony symbolizes that there is no separation. Elisabeth and Tom, of their own free will, have consciously chosen the awareness that they are one. The path that has made this a reality is their love for each other. Love knows no boundaries.

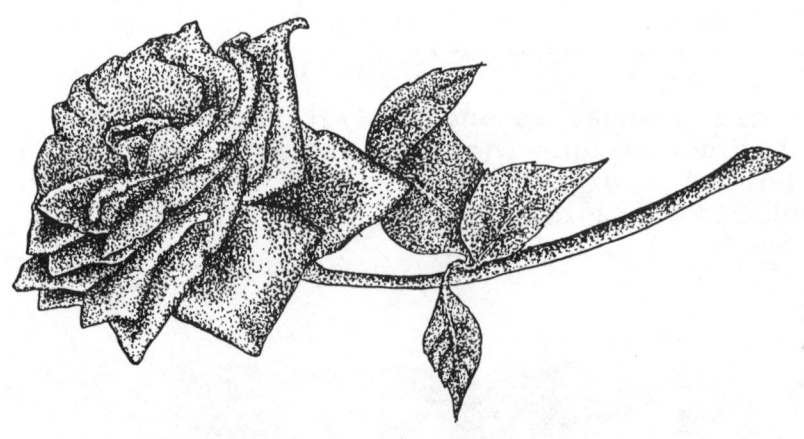

206

Brief Summary of the Wedding

The setting:

Set up crystal grid for the ceremony.

Music: Pachelbel's Canon. Tape and tape player

Smudge bride and groom

Opening prayers or readings

Attunement oils

Bride and groom enter the crystal grid

More readings on love and marriage

Consent / Vows

Blessing of the rings

Nuptial Blessing of the couple

Wedding Candle lighting (for indoor ceremony)

Tibetan Bells & Bowls

Reading: on Children

Circle of Children

Children Blessing the couple / parents

Crystal given to guests

Group Blessing

Wedding document signing for guests

Honeymoon candle (a white, six day votive candle)

Marriage Covenant

On this twenty-ninth day of May 1988 Berit Elisabeth Lindberg and Thomas Arthur Baldwin in the presence of God and these our friends, promise with Divine assistance to be unto each other, loving and faithful in the Covenant of Marriage so long as we both shall live.

_____
_____ Minister

And we, having been present at this Marriage as witnesses here unto set our hands.

_____   _____
_____   _____
_____   _____
_____   _____
_____   _____
_____   _____

- -

This document can be written in calligraphy on parchment paper or bristol board paper. I gave one to the wedding couple as a gift. An artist friend, Erica makes them. The document is very large (plus 14 " x 20 ") and it looks beautiful framed. The saying is based on a Quaker style wedding where the bride and groom marry each other. Be sure to tell Erica how many guests will be at the ceremony. She can make more signature lines if needed: Erica Risser Runkles, P.O. Box 37, West Willow, Pa. 17583

1. American Bible Society. <u>Good News Bible</u>. ABS, N.Y.C.,
   N.Y. 1976.

2. Gibran, Kahlil. <u>The Prophet</u>. Alfred Knopf, Inc., N.Y.C.,
   N.Y., 1923.

3. Yogananda, Paramahansa. A post card. Self-Realization
   Fellowship, 3880 San Rafael Ave., Los Angeles, Calif. 90065

4. Peter Pauper Press. <u>Love is a Poem</u>. Mt. Vernon, N.Y.,1962.

5. Mundy, Jon. <u>A Wedding Manual</u>. High Rock Graphics, 37 Hillside
   Terrace, Monroe, N.Y. 10950 $ 2.00.

6. The Standard Publishing Co. <u>A Christian Ministers Manual</u>.
   Cincinnati, Ohio, 1984.

   Other Related Books for this Chapter:

<u>The Book of Common Prayer</u>. The Church Hymnal Corp. and the Seabury
Press, 1977. It can be obtained through the Episcopal Church.

<u>The Rite of Marriage</u>. Catholic Book Publishing Co., N.Y.C.,
N.Y. 1970.

<u>Together for Life</u>. Ave Maria Press, Notre Dame, Indiana, 1970.

<u>A Complete Guide to All Religious Weddings & Interfaith Marriage
Services</u>. Abraham Klausner. Alpha Publishing Co.
ISBN # 0-933771-00-2.

Sources for Religious Supplies:

Holy Land Art Company
160 Chamber Street
N.Y.C., N.Y. 10007
(212) 962-2130

Barclay Church Supply
26 Warren Street
N.Y.C., N.Y. 10007
(212) 267-9432

Forrest Church Supply
Atlanta, Georgia

Send for their catalogs.

Look in the Yellow Pages for a religious supply store in your area.

Recommended Organizations:

The New Seminary
7 W. 96th St., Suite 19 B
N.Y.C., N.Y. 10025
(212) 866-3795

Certification training:

First Year students receive ordination and a certificate for Minister of Spiritual Counseling, M.S.C.

Second Year students belong to the School of Continuing Studies. They choose a field to specialize in such as: meditation, counseling or healing. Certification is given for Master of Spiritual Therapy, M.S.Th.

You will find that these are the only school certificates that have combined signatures of: a rabbi, a priest, a minister and a swami on them.

The New Seminary

School years begin every September and end in June. Students can take their training in person and attend classes twice a month, or they may choose to study by correspondence. There have been several students from different countries who have completed these programs.

The New Seminary offers either of these certifications upon successful completion of the school program. There is a mandatory intensive training, a review board and graduation attendance that is required for each enrolled student. Those who are interested in receiving a certificate for Master of Spiritual Therapy, may skip the first year of training. Not everyone is interested in becoming an ordained Interfaith Minister.

Second year training is open to graduates of any other seminary or spiritual institution. It is also open to those who have a practice in spiritual healing or counseling work. Applicants are required to obtain three letters of testimony regarding one's work in ministry, counseling or the healing arts.

Tuition - Contribution for the first year ministers' training is $ 1,000.00.

Tuition - Contribution for the second year spiritual therapists' training is $ 400.00.

Association of Interfaith Ministers
Village Station
P.O. Box 924
New York, N.Y. 10014-0924

Attention: Rev. Diane Kraus

Membership in this organization entitles one to possess a wallet size card identifying membership. This may or may not come in handy when doing hospital visits. AIM membership is available only to those who are ordained ministers. If you live in the N.Y. tri-state area, this organization offers various activities throughout the year.

COLOR   HEALING

and

CRYSTALS

Color Healing with Crystals

You can use crystals in Chromotherapy (color healing) session work.

The crystal can be programmed with a particular color. This can be done simply by thought. You can mentally project a particular color while holding a crystal in your hand for a few moments.

You can also use color gels and a light source (a light bulb or sunlight) and send the color vibration into the crystal. Some people do this for 5 - 15 minutes with a light / gel projection. If it is done with the gel and sun method, you may choose to program the crystal in this manner for fifteen minutes to an hour.

Healing Boxes: I know a man who is a stained glass craftsman. He makes small boxes out of stained glass. Some boxes are two or three colors. The inside bottom is a mirror. This can be used to return the vibrations that are projected onto it. The lid center piece is made with a clear quartz cluster or an amethyst cluster. The bottom of the cluster is exposed through the glass lid that surrounds it. Most people buy these boxes for their jewelry and trinkets.

You can use these healing boxes to charge objects: crystals, jewelry, healing objects, laser wands, etc. I use these boxes for absentee healing. I place a photo of a person inside the box. Sometimes, I place a small crystal or a cabochon on the photo. The box is then placed outside in the sun light. The lid is closed. The rays of the sun go through the stained glass and crystal cluster onto the photo inside. I always say a prayer that the healing serve the person to his / her highest good. Once the condition is set, my work is done.

You can use colored glass jars, bottles or goblets and fill them up with spring water. A quartz crystal can be placed into the water. Next, you can put the colored glass bottle outside in the sun. The sun will magnetize the water with its healing cosmic rays. The crystal in the water will amplify the charging process. This method can be done for anywhere from fifteen minutes to a full afternoon. A good average time is one hour.

You can also program crystals with color for chakra balance work. See my book, <u>Crystal Therapeutics</u>.

Each chakra is balanced with one or two particular color vibrations. Here is a list of colors used for balancing various imbalances:

RED: Blood disorders, lack of vitality, paralysis, poor circulation, anemia, colds, impotence.

Always follow this color with green or blue before ending the treatment.

ORANGE: Spleen infections, kidney diseases, bronchitis, paralysis, gallstones, circulation, gas and digestion problems, bone development, asthma, overcome fear, bronchitis, epilepsy, cholera, cessation of menstruation, colon disorders, menstrual cramps, depression, mononucleosis.

This color recharges the etheric body.

YELLOW: For imbalances in the liver, intestines, digestion problems, skin disorders, diabetes (pancreas), mental and nervous exhaustion, dyspepsia, flatulence, constipation, stomach troubles, indigestion, heartburn, paralysis, eczema, leprosy, depression, mental stimulant, colitis, hepatitis, lack of appetite, gall bladder, nervous breakdown, strokes.

Do not us this color for diarrhea or acute inflammations.

GREEN: Emotional problems, heart and blood pressure disorders, cancer, nervous system, tired nerves, master tonic, headaches, ulcers, neuralgia, influenza, syphilis, jaundice, muscular dystrophy and muscle rebuilding, tissue rebuilder, tumors, dissolves blood clots.

BLUE: For infectious diseases, hysteria, insomnia, most inflammations, headaches, spasms, fevers, burns, irritations, laryngitis, colic, skin abrasions, jaundice, teething, throat disorders, rheumatism, sciatica, diarrhea, hysteria, rabies, neuritis, epilepsy, bronchitis, pleurisy, hemorrhages, cramps, endo and myocarditis, gonorrhea, abscesses, carcinoma, bursitis, infections, shingles, measles, nausea, nose bleeds, sun stroke, stress, high blood pressure, pain, cystitis.

INDIGO: Eyes, ear and nose.   Also for asthma, bronchitis, pneumonia, deafness, cataracts, eye inflammations, excitable or violent mental states, nosebleed, diphtheria, nervous irritation, insomnia, exorcism, facial paralysis, glaucoma, hemorrhage, tuberculosis.

VIOLET: For stress, insomnia, cataracts, neurosis, neuralgic headache, epilepsy, spinal meningitis, reduces appetite, cerebral disease, cancer, diarrhea, concussion, gonorrhea, sciatica.

This is a very fast vibration.   Do not use it for a long length of time.   It is not for undeveloped minds or retardation.

PINK: This is the universal color of unconditional love.   It balances the heart chakra and is used for emotional healing.

      There are many wonderful books on the subject of color healing.   Here is a list of my favorites:

Colour Healing by Mary Anderson

The Power of the Rays by S.G.J. Ouseley

The Seven Keys to Color Healing by Roland Hunt

Seven Mansions of Color by Alex Jones

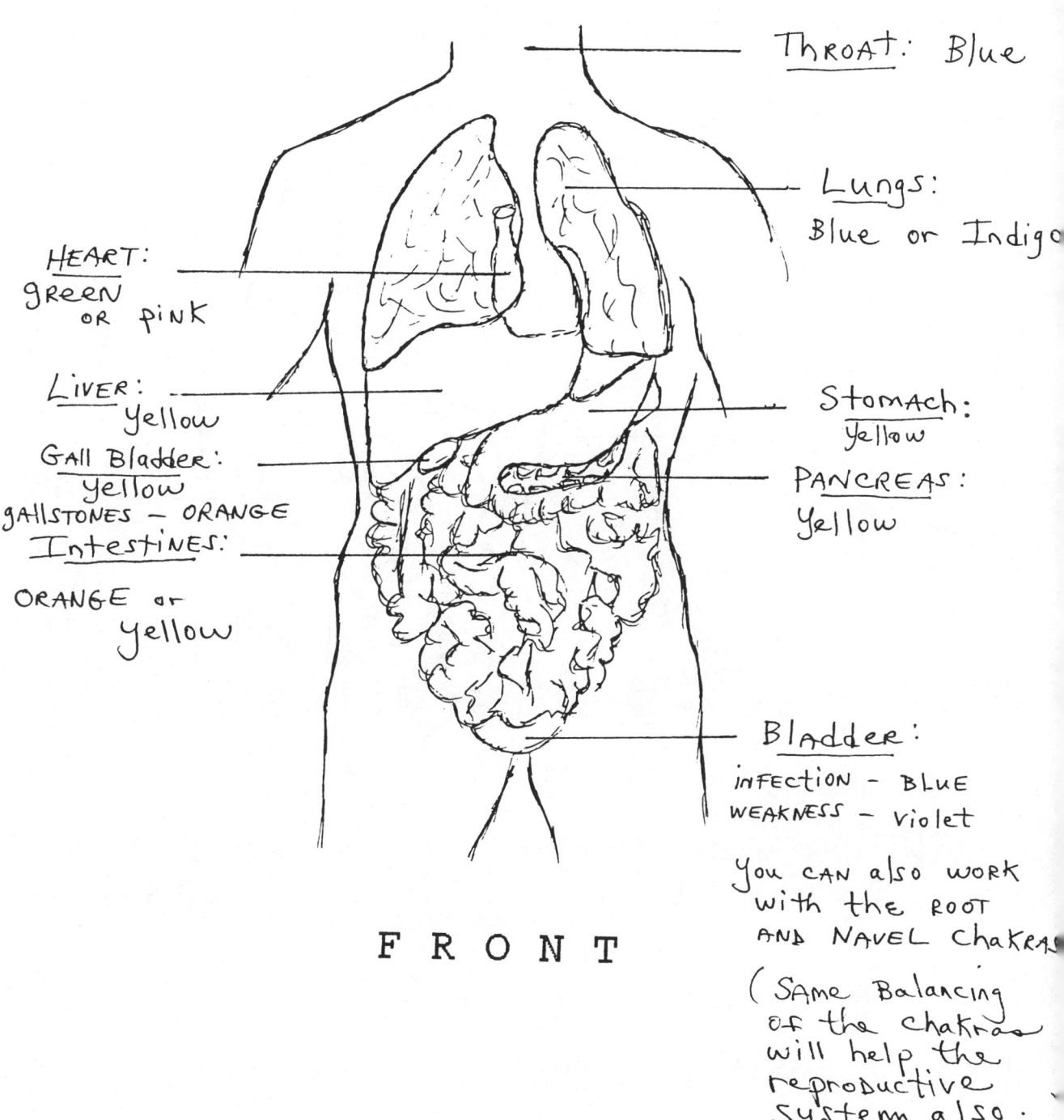

THROAT: Blue

Lungs:
Blue or Indigo

HEART:
green or pink

LIVER:
Yellow

GAll Bladder:
Yellow
gAllstones — ORANGE

Intestines:

ORANGE or
Yellow

Stomach:
Yellow

PANCREAS:
Yellow

Bladder:
iNfeCTiON — BLUE
WEAKNESS — violet

You cAN also work
with the Root
AND NAVEL chakRA

(SAme Balancing
of the chakras
will help the
reproductive
System also.

F R O N T

217

COLOR ASSOCIATIONS for BALANCING

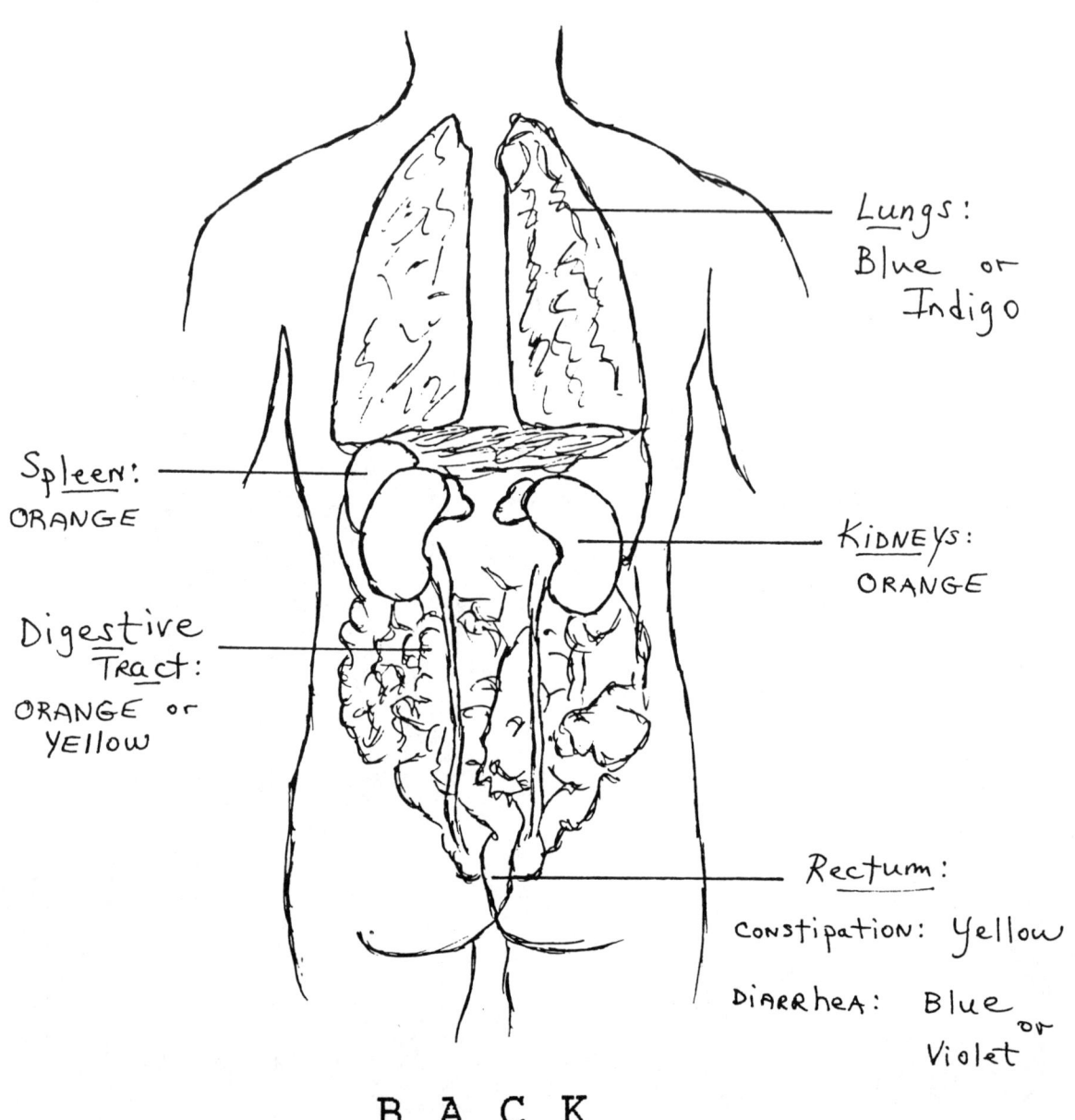

Lungs:
Blue or
Indigo

Spleen:
ORANGE

Kidneys:
ORANGE

Digestive
Tract:
ORANGE or
Yellow

Rectum:

Constipation: Yellow

Diarrhea: Blue or
Violet

B A C K

Sedona and the Stars, Moon with a Ring

2/88

Starlit path
Spiritual journey
Child of God
Walking in Light
Becoming Light
Being a Light
Being.... knowingness.

Keeper of the Flame
Wisdom of Spirit
Spiritual wisdom
Guardian of shared secrets
Support on the journey
Guide us well.

Lover of Love
Love expression
Heart opener
Expanding energy force
Teach and share with us
the Love vibration.

As we sense this...

We envelop in Love.
We become Love.
We are the Love expression
Sharing this within and without.

As Love emanates,
It is happily contagious.

All are in Spirit expression.
All are Love.
All are Light.
All are Peace.

We are all consciousness
Sharing
and becoming One,
Becoming Whole.

We are God.

ABOUT THE AUTHOR

REV. OJELA FRANK, M.S.C., M.S.Th. has been active in holistic health and the healing arts for eighteen years. She has traveled extensively throughout the United States and has studied many healing modalities including: Therapeutic Touch, Guided Imagery, Thymo-Kinesiology, Crystal Healing, Advanced Reiki Healing, Shantira and MariEl Healing, to name a few. Ojela is an ordained Interfaith Minister and a graduate of the New Seminary in New York City. She is Director of the Holistic Health Works, which offers counseling and healing therapies. Ojela is President of Spiritual Awareness Dynamics, Inc., which offers training programs in the healing arts. Her main focus is energy balancing, counseling and teaching her clients and students how to relax and open up to their true expressions. Ojela is author of <u>Crystal Therapeutics</u> and founder of the Crystal Therapeutics training seminars.

BIBLIOGRAPHY

Alper, Frank. Exploring Atlantis Vol. II & III. Thousand Oaks, Ca. : Quantum Productions, 1981 & 1982.

American Bible Society. Good News Bible. New York, N.Y.: ABS, 1977.

Anderson, Mary. Colour Healing. Wellingborough, Northamptonshire, Gr. Britain: The Aquarian Press, 1979.

Babitt, Edwin. The Principles of Light and Color. Secaucus, N.J.: Citadel Press, 1967.

Blackburn, Gabriele. The Science and Art of the Pendulum. Ojai, Ca.: Idylwild Books, 1983.

Bynner, Witter. The Way of Life According to Lao Tzu. New York, N.Y.: Capricorn Books, 1962.

Drake, Stanley. The Path to Birth. Edinburgh, Gr. Britain: Floris Books, 1979.

Finch, Elizabeth & Bill. Photo-chromotherapy. Phoenix, Az.: Esoterica Publications, 1972. (out of print)

Frank, Ojela. Crystal Therapeutics. New City, N.Y.: The Holistic Health Works, 1987.

Gibran, Kahlil. The Prophet. New York City, N.Y.: Alfred Knopf, Inc., 1923.

Hay, Louise. Heal Your Body. Santa Monica, Ca.: Hay House, 1982.

Hunt, Roland. The Seven Rays of Color Healing. San Francisco, Ca.: Harper & Row, 1971.

International Committee on English in Liturgy, Inc. Rite of Baptism for Children. New York City, N.Y.: Catholic Book Publishing Co., 1969.

Jones, Alex. Seven Mansions of Color. Marina del Rey, Ca.: DeVorss & Co., 1982.

Keyes, Ken. Handbook to Higher Consciousness. Coos Bay, Or.: Ken Keyes College, 1975.

Krum, Carol. Reiki Healing Workshops, 1985.

Mariechild, Diane. Mother Wit. Trumansburg, N.Y.: The Crossing Press, 1981.

Mundy, Jon. A Wedding Manual. Monroe, N.Y.: High Rock Graphics.

Ouseley, S.G.J. The Power of the Rays. Romford, Essex, Gr. Britain: L.N. Fowler & Co. Ltd., 1983.

Peace, Crystal. Quartz Crystals and Other Gemstones. Rte. 2 Box 240A, Clyde, N.C. 28721, 1984.

Peter Pauper Press. Love Is a Poem. Mt. Vernon, N.Y., 1962.

Peterson, Serenity. Crystal Visioning. Nashville, Tenn.: Interdimensional Pub., 1984.

Research, Health. Color Healing. Mokelumne Hill, Ca.: Health Research, 1956.

The Standard Publishing Co. A Christian Ministers Manual. Cincinnati, Ohio, 1984.

Tortora and Anagnostakos. Principles of Anatomy and Physiology. New York City, N.Y.: Harper & Row, 1981.

ADVANCED   TRAINING

in   the

HEALING   ARTS

Where Do I Go from Here?

Healing Arts Resource Guide:

Schools and Programs for Advanced Training

Crystal Therapeutics
P.O. Box 596, Dept. B
Bardonia, N.Y. 10954

National Seminars and certification training: Offers seven levels
of training, including two teacher certifications. Crystal
Therapeutics is a division of Spiritual Awareness Dynamics, Inc.,
which also offers other training programs. Send a postage stamp
with a request for a current class schedule or a sponsor packet
for workshops in your area.

Arizona Metaphysical Society
P.O. Box 44027
Phoenix, Az.   85064

Dr. Frank Alper offers Carousel of Growth Seminars on an international level.   These are wonderful spiritual development
workshops. Advanced training leads to certification as a healer-
counselor or a minister in an international church. Dr. Alper is
a famous channel who also does private " soul life " readings.
(At this present time, he is the best channeler who has ever done
a reading for me.)   Write for Dr. Alper's current travel
schedule.

The New Seminary
7 West 96th St., Suite 19 B
New York City, N.Y. 10025

One to two year certification training as an Ordained Interfaith
Minister or a Master of Spiritual Therapy. Training is offered
locally or you can study by correspondence and then come to the
mandatory three day intensive at the end of the school year.
School year begins September and ends in June. Write for a free
brochure.

The Reiki Alliance
P.O. Box 41   (new address)
Cataldo, Idaho   83810

The Reiki Alliance supports Phyllis Lei Furumoto as the Reiki
Grandmaster and offers international training seminars. It
offers certification training for practitioners and teachers
(Reiki Masters). It advertises mostly by word of mouth. I
support it fully and want to let you know about this group.
Phyllis also has been offering a wonderful week long seminar on
emotional healing for several years. It is called a " Self-
assessment " workshop. It is open to anyone who has taken
training in Reiki at any level. I found it to be one of the most
awakening experiences in my life. Thank you, Phyllis! Keep up
the good work.

Center of the Light
P.O. Box 540
Great Barrington, Mass.   01230

Eva and Eugene Graf are founders of this healing school. It
offers a two year certification training in the healing arts. It
is a very well rounded program. Many commute from quite a
distance to take this training. Classes are held one weekend a
month for two years. The center is nicely located in the country
and also offers weekend workshops throughout the summer with
several gifted instructors. Write for a free brochure of summer
workshops.

Omega Institute
Lake Drive
R.D. 2 Box 377
Rhinebeck, N.Y.   12572

Summer camp: What better way to spend a part of the summer?
Omega has been offering training in the healing arts, arts,
meditation and holistic health for over ten years. You can choose
from a fantastic schedule of week long or weekend seminars with
some of the best and famous teachers in the world. It is a
rewarding experience. Write for a free brochure of summer events.

The Open Center
83 Spring St.
New York City, N.Y.   10012

You have to be in the area to enjoy this jewel. They also get
some of the best teachers. Classes are offered on a week night
or weekend basis all year long. Write for a seasonal brochure of
events.   The center also offers interesting group tours to
different parts of the world.

Interface
552 Main St.
Watertown, Mass.   02171

This is a similar set up like the N.Y. Open Center, but it is
located in the Boston area. A good variety of classes for week
nights and weekends. Write for a current schedule of events.

Metaphysical Center of New Jersey
P.O. Box 94
Bloomingdale, N.J.   07403

This is probably the only group in the country that offers a
twelve semester course of study in metaphysics and parapsychology
in an adult education program. Classes are taught at public
schools. This group has done much to introduce " New Age "
thought to the mainstream. This organization has been active
since 1956! It also offers monthly lectures and workshops with
well known guest speakers. Sometimes, it offers an annual weekend
seminar with famous speakers and draws a large crowd for this
event. If you live in the N.Y. tri-state area, write for a
schedule of events.

New Age Center
1-3 So. Broadway
Nyack, N.Y.   10960

I have taught here for four years. It is a nice little place that
offers a large selection of workshops and classes. Every season
is active. Dr. Ken Pollinger is the director. He is open to new
guest lecturers. It's a good place to start out for teaching.
Write for a brochure of events.

Wise Woman Center
P.O. Box 64
Woodstock, N.Y.   12498

Susun Weed, the author of the <u>Wise Woman Herbal for the Childbearing Year</u> offers training in herbs and healing. Her center is open mostly from Spring through Fall. Susun also travels and teaches throughout the world. Write for her brochure of workshops.

Kripalu Center for Yoga & Health
Box 793
Lenox, Mass.   02140

This is one of the best health centers in the country. Come to experience the community. Guru Amrit Desai is the founder of this center.   Initially it was located in Pennsylvania, but its popularity outgrew the smaller center. A beautiful setting with mountains and a private lake is yours to behold. The center offers certification training for yoga instructors and various healing arts. Pamper yourself with polarity therapy and bodywork with the gifted practitioners. I call Amrit Desai the funny guru. He has a warm sense of humor in his teachings. Enjoy. The center has a brochure with seasonal training programs and a product catalog. It also offers residential work / study programs.

Life Spectrums   (Northeast)
P.O. Box 373
Harrisburg, Pa.   17108
                                    or

Carol Tucker, Register
2177 Lincoln Ave. # 18   (Canada)
Montreal, Quebec
CANADA H3H1J2

I mentioned this one and some of the other ones in my previous book. They are worth mentioning again. Each summer for one week around July 4th, this group offers a week long seminar in Elizabethtown, Penna. The seminar draws people from all over the country.   Some of the speakers are famous and the energy of everyone coming together is fantastic.   It offers a healing service at the end of the week. It is a very special experience to watch twenty to thirty healers and workshop speakers offer free healings to a group of three to four hundred people. You can write for a seminar brochure.

Spiritual Frontier Fellowship
10819 Winner Road   (national
Independence, Mo. 64052-0519   headquarters)

Diane Downer, Register
167 Warren Way   (Northeast)
Lancaster, Pa. 17601

C.P. 1445 Stn. " H "
Montreal, Quebec   (Canada)
CANADA H3G2N3

This group has seminars throughout the country. At the
Elizabethtown Retreat, it is usually back to back with the Life
Spectrum seminar. Many famous teachers offer a week long
workshop. At the local level, the group offers lectures on a
monthly basis. You can become a member of this organization by
writing to the address in Missouri. It will refer you to a local
chapter in your area.

Women's Herbalist's Conference
Collette Gardiner, Finance Coordinator
Women's Herbalist Conference
P.O. Box 1510
Jacksonville, Oregon 97539

The top female herbalists of the country gather to share with
other women. The weekend workshop is attended by women from all
over the country. Write for the next scheduled dates.

Medicine Wheel Gatherings
The Bear Tribe Medicine Society
Box 9167   attn: Singing
Spokane, Wash. 99209   Pipe Woman

Native American traditionalists share with others. The Bear Tribe
also offers apprenticeships with Sun Bear at its center and across
the nation. It also offers the experience of Sweat Lodges and
Vision Quests. Write for the scheduled events for Spring through
Fall. The Bear Tribe goes to different regions of the country.
Medicine people from various tribes come to share their wisdom.
We thank you, Sun Bear.

Rowe Conference Center
Kings Highway Road
Rowe, Mass. 01367

This center offers workshops with famous teachers Spring through
Fall. Write for a list of the workshops.

The Academy of Mantura Arts & Sciences
P.O. Box 58098
Renton, Wash.   98058

National seminars in ancient healing arts of: Shantira, Kofutu Touch Healing and Venkara Crystals - Mantras. Shantira Healing is for personal chakra work. It can also be used on others and for distant healing. Kofutu is another healing method that has several levels of training based on " laying of hands " and the use of sacred energy symbols. Write for a brochure of current workshops.

Sunray Meditation Society
Rd. 1 Box 87
Huntington, Vt.   05462

I first met Dhyani Ywahoo at a lecture in Boulder, Colorado in 1982. I will never forget her. Dhyani is a Cherokee Medicine Woman who carries the lineage of her tradition. She shares Native American teachings and teaches the Peacekeeper Mission throughout the country. Dhyani's teachings come from her heart. She is a very special woman. Her voice is very powerful when she sings her native chants. You can write for her teaching schedules and audio tapes at the above address. I highly recommend experiencing Dhyani. Many major cities now have centers that explore her teachings. Look in your local New Age newspapers. Dhyani has just written a book, <u>Voices of Our Ancestors</u>. I suggest you get it.

Barbara Brennan
331 E. 71st St. Box 21
N.Y.C., N.Y.   10021

Barbara Brennan is the author of <u>Hands of Light</u>. It is one of the best books I've ever come across on healing. Barbara's center offers a four year training course in the healing arts. Write for the training program information and Barbara's teaching schedule.

RESOURCE   GUIDE

to

NEW   AGE   CENTERS

MORE TRAINING CENTERS

Aloha International
P.O. Box 665   (Kahuna teachings)
Kilauea, Hawaii 96754

Brugh Joy, Inc.
P.O. Box 895
Lucerne Valley, Ca. 92356

Wainwright House
Center for Development of Human Resources
260 Stuyvesant Ave.
Rye, N.Y. 10580

Sufi Healing Order
Rt. 2 Box 166
Leicester, N.C. 28748

Naropa Institute
2130 Arapahoe
Boulder, Co. 80302

Integrative Studies Institute
Box 2349 B
Cambridge, Mass. 02238

Holistic Health Assoc.
of the Princeton Area
360 Nassau St.
Princeton, N.J. 08540

Unison Learning Center
68 Mtn. Rest Rd.
New Paltz, N.Y. 12561

Himalayan Institute
Rd. 1 Box 88
Honesdale, Pa. 18431

American Institute of Metaphysical Studies
2000 L. Street NW Suite 200
Washington, D.C. 20036

The Rubenfeld Center
115 Waverly Place
New York, N.Y. 10011

Healing Light Center
Rosalin Bryere
204 E. Wilson St.
Glendale, Ca.   90206

Healing Tao Center   (National)
P.O. Box 1194
Huntington, N.Y. 11743

MariEl Healing Training
Ethel Lombardi   (National)
93 Spring Creek Rd.   Rt. 5
Lockport, Ill.   60441

Dr. Jay Scherer's
Academy of Natural Healing
320 E. Marcy
Santa Fe, N.M.   87501

Traditional Medicine Conference
Fernald Center
P.O. Box 698
Springville, Ca.   93265

Institute of Mental Physics
P.O. Box 640
Yucca Valley, Ca.   92284

Acupressure - Acupuncture Institute
7875 Bird Road
Miami, Florida   33155

Dechen Yonten Dzo Institute
of Buddhist Medicine
1775 Linden Ave.
Boulder, Co.   80302

P.H.D.
449 Pemberwick Rd.
Western Greenwich Civic Center
Greenwich, Ct.   06830

Potomac Myotherapy Institute
7826 Eastern Ave.   NW
Washington, D.C.   20012

The Lively Stones Fellowship
Rev. Willard Fuller
P.O. Box 2007
Palatka, Florida   32078

New Mexico School of Natural Therapeutics
117 Richmond N.E.
Albuquerque, N.M.   87106

American Institute of Hypnotherapy
1805 E. Garry, Suite 100
Santa Ana, Ca.   92705

American College of Nutripathy
6821 East Thomas Rd.
Scottsdale, Az.   85251

Heartwood Institute
220 Harmony Lane
Garberville, Ca.   95440

Institute of Psycho-Structural Balancing
4501 Cass St.
San Diego, Ca.   92109

California Institute
of Integral Studies
765 Ashbury St.
San Francisco, Ca.   94117

Body Electric School of Massage and Rebirthing
6527 A Telegraph Ave.
Oakland, Ca.   94609

The New Mexico Academy of Massage
and Advanced Healing Arts
P.O. Box 932
Santa Fe, N.M.   87504

Dallas Professional Massage Studies
3611 McKinney Ave. # 110
Dallas, Tx.   75204

     Please refer to my book, <u>Crystal Therapeutics</u> for a list of
more New Age centers. The third edition of this book has a new
extended mailing list.

ORDER FORM

	Price	Quan.	Amount
Books			
Crystal Therapeutics ^{SM} by Rev. Ojela Frank	$15.95	_____	_____
Advanced Crystal Therapeutics ^{SM} by Rev. Ojela Frank	$18.95	_____	_____
Instructional Cassettes			
Crystal Healing: A Beginner's Workshop (Two Tape Set)	$18.00	_____	_____
Healing Ourselves and Our Emotions	$9.95	_____	_____
Discount Product Catalog			
Retail or Wholesale (Circle One)	$1.00	_____	_____

Sub-total _____

N.Y. residents add 6.25% tax _____

Add $1.00 shipping per item _____
(except catalog only)

Grand Total _____

(Allow 2 -6 weeks for delivery from deposit of check.)

Make check payable to: Holistic Health Works
P.O. Box 327
New City, New York 10956

To:

Holistic Health Works
P. O. Box 327 - bc
New City, N. Y. 10956

From:

_____

_____

☐ I would like to be on your mailing list.

☐ I would like to receive a catalog of your books, tapes, crystals and jewelry.

☐ I would like information on your workshops, classes in the Crystal Therapeutics[SM] program.

☐ Please send me a sponsor packet so we can sponsor a workshop in our area.

☐ I would like to order the following (see reverse side).